A PRACTIC
ILLUSTRATED GUIDE
TO
MODERN ORTHOPAEDICS

Alexander Carlos, Orthopaedic Technologist

Thank you:
Dr. Gordon Dale, Orthopaedic Surgeon
Dion Maxwell, R. T. Orthopaed
Charles Mellish, R. T. Orthopaed
Peter Grice, R. T. Orthopaed
Ron Wallace, R. T. Orthopaed
Brian Abdul, R. T. Orthopaed
Canadian Society of Orthopaedic Technologists (C.S.O.T.)
National Association of Orthopaedic Technologists (N.A.O.T.)
Career Canada College
St. Michael's Hospital, Toronto
St. Joseph's Hospital, Toronto
Selected illustrations and text on Traction Guidelines (chapter 9)
reproduced from the Zimmer Traction Handbook© 2004,
Zimmer Orthopaedic Surgical Products, Inc.
Ray Eusebio, Los Angeles
To my students, past and present
Illustrations by Bernardo Sembrano
Design & layout by AdamsonGraphics.net
Typing by Barbara-Lynn Adamson

ISBN 978-1-896616-05-6

Printed in USA.

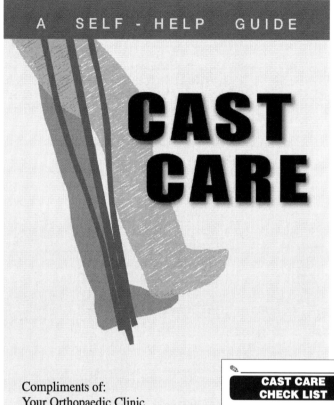

A SELF - HELP GUIDE

CAST CARE

Compliments of:
Your Orthopaedic Clinic
76 Main St.
Your City, State
Tel: 555.555.5555

- 68 pages 5.25" x 7"
- Cast Care Checklist
- Warning Signs
- Interactive Sections
- Easy To Read
  (Reader's Digest Format)
- Crutches & Exercises Explained
- Helps Remove Fear
  and Misunderstanding
- Mainstream - Not Controversial
- Legally & Medically Approved
- Self Help and Self Care Tips
- Low Price (less than $2.00)
  Volume Discounts Available

Free Imprint on Front Cover

CAST CARE CHECK LIST

	Yes	No
Did the cast dry properly?	☐	☐
Do I know the type of cast material?	☐	☐
Do I know how to clean the cast?	☐	☐
Do I always keep the cast dry?	☐	☐
Do I know how to repair/smooth the rough edges on the cast?	☐	☐
Do I know not to scratch inside the cast?	☐	☐
Do I know how to prevent swelling by elevation?	☐	☐
Do I know how to use crutches properly?	☐	☐
Do I know the warning signs when to phone the doctor?	☐	☐

Hopefully you have answered "yes" to all these questions.

59

Color Tear-Off Cast Care Checklist Available

- SAVE TIME
- HELP AVOID LITIGATION ISSUES
- ENSURE PATIENT COMPLIANCE
- PROMOTE YOUR CLINIC

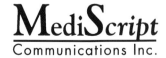
MediScript
Communications Inc.

Contains:
- Information for caregiver and patient.
- Helps avoid litigation issues.
- Comprehensive prevention tips.
- All treatment options explained.
- Pressure redistribution devices.
- Interactive progress charts & checklists.

Other Wound Care Titles:
- Diabetic Foot Ulcers
- Venous Leg Ulcers
- Burn Care
- Incontinence Care
- Living With a Colostomy
- Living With an Ileostomy
- Living With a Urostomy
- Healing Wounds Successfully
- Diabetes and Feet

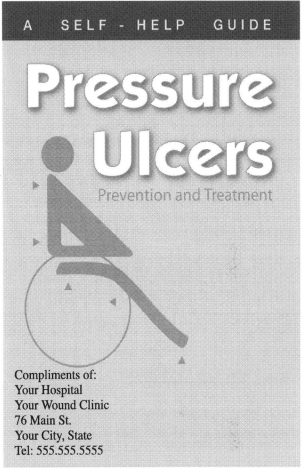

A SELF - HELP GUIDE

Pressure Ulcers

Prevention and Treatment

Compliments of:
Your Hospital
Your Wound Clinic
76 Main St.
Your City, State
Tel: 555.555.5555

Free Imprint on Front Cover

MediScript
Communications Inc.
www.mediscript.net

Contact us at:
Email - mediscript30@yahoo.ca
Tel - 800.773.5088
Fax - 800.639.3186
We will send you a free sample

Mediscript Communications Inc., the publisher has designed this book to provide information to the subject matter covered. It is sold with the understanding that the publisher and author and contributors are not liable for the misconception or misuse of information provided. Every effort has been made to make this book as complete and accurate as possible. The purpose of this book is to educate, visually clarify and provide a reference guide to the subject of orthopaedics. It is an informal learning adjunct to the material you have from courses you have attended and officially recommended text books. Consequently the publisher, author and contributors shall have neither liability or responsibility to any person or entity with respect to any loss, damage, failed examinations or injury caused or alleged to be caused by the information contained within this book. The information presented herein is in no way intended as a substitute for medical teachers or other medical text books.

Library of Congress Cataloging – in – Publication Data
Alexander Carlos
Modern Orthopaedics / by Alexander Carlos
Includes bibliographic references
ISBN 1 – 55040 – 056 – 8
1. Orthopaedics 2. Modern Orthopaedics 3. Casting 4. Fractures -
   Classification   5. Fractures – Types 6. Traction – Guidelines

How to order more copies of this book

Regular single copy price US $19.95. Quantity discounts available.
mediscript30@yahoo.ca
Tel 800 773 5088
Fax 800 639 3186 for North America
Tel. for International customers:
North America code Tel. (519) 823 1769 Fax (519) 341 9319
Website www.mediscript .net

Other (patient education) books from Mediscript

ABOUT THE AUTHOR

Alexander Carlos was first registered as an Orthopaedic Technologist in 1984 and during his career he has been a college instructor in orthopaedics and an international orthopaedic manufacturer's consultant. During his time as an instructor he saw a need for a "down to earth" guide book for modern orthopaedics for a wide-ranging audience of health care practitioners. Alex is very much a "people" person and was able to harness the efforts of many professionals in producing this book.

Most importantly, Alex had the vision to see the importance of the hand drawn anatomical diagrams and recruited a talented medical illustrator, Bernard Sembrano, to produce these drawings under Alex's leadership. These quality illustrations are pivotal to the success of the book.

From his own notes, manufacturers' educational aids, physician and surgeon involvement, student feedback, suggestions from fellow orthopaedic technologists and technicians, and research into the basics of modern orthopaedics, Alex has produced this highly acclaimed and unique book.

TABLE OF CONTENTS

Introduction 9

Chapter One - Anatomical Terminology 11

Chapter Two - The Skeletal System 23
Bones 24
Differences between a man's and a woman's skeleton 31
Cartilage 33
Joints...34
Illustrations – *Skeletal System, 38 *Skull, 40 *Pelvis, 43
*Vertebral Column, 44 *Humerus, 45 *Radius and Ulna,46
*Femur, 47 *Patella, 47 *Tibia/Fibula, 48 *Foot, 49 *Hand, 51

Chapter Three - The Muscular System 53
Muscle structure..54
Muscle contraction...55
Functions of the skeletal muscle..58
Specific muscles and actions...61
Illustrations – *Skin Structure, 56 *Muscular System, 69
*Achilles' Tendon, 71 *Rotator Cuff, 72 *Quadriceps, 73 *Hamstring, 74

Chapter Four – Casting 75
History 76
Cast setting 76
Equipment used in casting..79
Types of cast immobilization 83

Chapter Five - Cast Complications 87

Chapter Six – Types and Classifications of Fractures.................93

Chapter Seven - Upper Extremity Fractures 133
Colles...134
Scaphoid 137
Bennet's...139
Boxer's 140
Humerus 141
Clavicle 144

Chapter Eight - Lower Extremity Fractures 145
Hip..146
Femur 148
Patella..151
Knee 152
Tibia..153
Tarsal 156
Metatarsal...157

Table of Contents Continued

Chapter Nine - Traction Guidelines 159
General information..160
Types of traction...163
Application of traction 169
Principles of traction 172
Contraindications to skin traction 175
Complications 175
Bradford frame and Thomas splint..177
Slings and springs...180
Gallow's traction (Bryant's)...182
Cervicle traction 184
Traction on the humerus..187
Pelvic traction with pelvic belt..191
Buck's traction..194
Leg traction using Böhler-Braun frame 198
Russel's traction..201
Split Russel's traction...203
Thomas or Brady leg splint 204

Glossary of Roots and Suffixes..207

References Cited and Bibliography..209

Introduction

This book is meant to satisfy a variety of needs for all people involved directly or indirectly with the medical practice of orthopaedics.

For those who are studying to pass examinations in the subject of orthopaedics or who are trying to become a registered or certified orthopaedic technologist or technician, this book can be looked upon as a learning adjunct resource. You will have the curriculum guidelines for your course, recommended text books, and will have attended many practical sessions as well as have other written material from manufacturers, journals and seminar notes.

Modern Orthpaedics, however, can be looked upon as a great "leveler", containing as it does the basic facts and illustrations, presented in an accessible, inexpensive, forthright and friendly manner.

Medical text books can be expensive, voluminous and sometimes a little overwhelming; **Modern Orthopaedics** is just the opposite. A practical, easy to use reference guide, this book provides guidance principles, definitions and, most importantly, a fresh, illuminating visual depiction of the healthy and also demised anatomy. All the illustrations are hand drawn in a way that depicts the essence of the anatomical structure. They show you the critical aspects of the vulnerable skeletal structures and can provide the first stepping stone for diagnosis, understanding and treatment action.

Think of the drawings and content as a draft blueprint on which you can proceed with the confidence of understanding and insight. At the very least, **Modern Orthopaedics** can be a catalyst for seeking further information, talking to a colleague, taking further patient diagnostic tests, or provide help in clarifying a situation.

Every country has its own particular health model for the practice of orthopaedics; we like to think this book is an educational common denominator, crossing cultural and job description boundaries. After all, a broken bone has to be treated, irrespective of whether the medical person is a nurse, orthopaedic assistant, orthopaedic technologist, general practitioner, orthopaedic technician, physicians assistant, orthopaedic surgeon or rural physician.

The principles of treatment are the same, even though techniques or products used can differ.

In fact, there are a great many types of health care professionals who can practice orthopaedics. In the US, anybody appointed by an orthopaedic surgeon can apply a cast. In isolated rural areas, out of necessity, any qualified health care professional can practice basic orthopaedics. Various health care models dictate that for convenience for the patient and various economic factors, orthopaedics can be carried out in a general practitioner's office. The introduction of "surgi centers" for efficient and convenient access for patient treatment widens the spectrum of people practicing orthopaedics.

A further dimension is the constructive role health care product manufacturers play in educating and training health care professionals. The use of key products, from instruments and equipment for complex orthopaedic operations, to actual casting supplies for basic fractures, are all areas for manufacturers' involvement as part of the medical team.

For the beginner studying orthopaedics, this book can be a useful introductory aid, providing all the key terms, with explanations and visual depictions of anatomy and injuries.

For the established orthopaedic practitioner, this book can not only be a useful mind jogger but one to recommend to your colleagues in order to familiarize them with the basics of your specialty. In the end, **Modern Orthopaedics** can save you time and improve the medical team's treatment activities.

We have found it useful to divide the content into simple, short chapter categories enabling quick and easy reference and eliminating the need for an index.

As a final note, this book has been written keeping in mind at all times a vital corollary to the successful practice of modern orthopaedics: the importance of patient education as a tool for enhancing patient compliance to treatment. In the field of post-operative orthopaedic treatment, the patient's understanding of warning signs and self care practices can be an integral part of an optimum health outcome.

It is all too easy – especially in the practice of orthpaedics, which generally focuses on a specific injured skeletal body part – to look upon the patient as an object. The bone is broken, it has to be fixed. However, effective communication to the patient coupled with a patient education brochure or booklet to reinforce your message can be an invaluable aid to doing justice to your skilled treatment activities.

This book is essentially a collaborative effort from orthopaedic technologists and technicians, orthopaedic surgeons, nurses, instructors and physicians. It has been reviewed by a wide variety of medical practitioners and subsequently fine tuned in order to produce an affordable, practical publication that, we hope, fills a critical, unique need in the field of modern orthopaedics.

CHAPTER 1
ANATOMICAL
TERMINOLOGY

Anatomical Planes and Sections

When internal anatomy is described, the body or an organ is often cut or sectioned in a specific way so as to make particular structures easily visible. A **plane** is an imaginary flat surface that separates two portions of the body or an organ.

Frontal (coronal) section: A plane from side to side separates the body into front and back portions.

Sagittal section: A plane from front to back separates the body into right and left portions. A midsagittal section creates equal right and left halves.

Transverse section: A horizontal plane separates the body into upper and lower portions.

Cross section: A plane perpendicular to the long axis of an organ. A cross section of the small intestine (which is a tube) would look like a circle with the cavity of the intestine in the center.

Longitudinal section: A plane along the long axis of an organ. A frontal section of the **femur** (thigh bone) would also be a longitudinal section.

Axis: The central line around which a structure, pattern or figure is built or formed (a main stem or central cylinder).

Perpendicular: Forming an angle of 90° with another line, plane or surface.

Horizontal: Right angle to a radius of the earth.

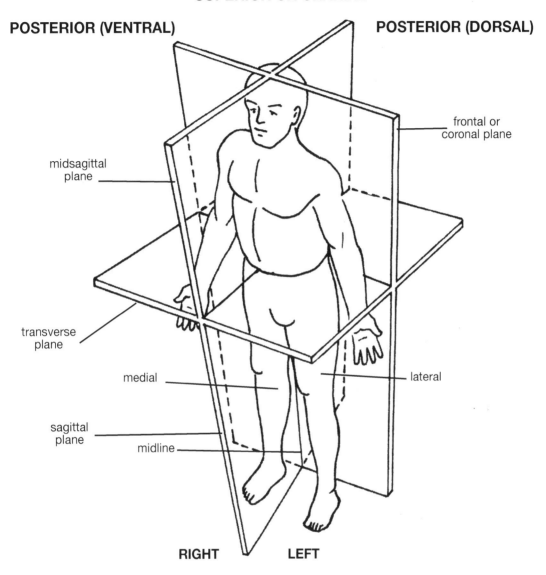

SUPERIOR OR CRANIAL

POSTERIOR (VENTRAL)

POSTERIOR (DORSAL)

frontal or
coronal plane

midsagittal
plane

transverse
plane

medial

lateral

sagittal
plane

midline

RIGHT

LEFT

INFERIOR OR CAUDAL

BODY PLANES AND SECTIONS

Skeletal Divisions

1: Head (cephalic)
2: Skull (cranial)
3: Face (facial)
4: Neck (cervical)
5: Forehead (frontal)
6: Eye (orbital)
7: Cheek (buccal)
8: Nose (nasal)
9: Mouth (oral)
10: Chest (thoracic)
11: Armpit (axillary)
12: Arm (brachial)
13: Front of elbow
    (antecubital)
14: Navel (umbilical)
15: Forearm (antebrahial)
16: Pelvis: (pelvic)
17: Groin (inguinal)
18: Wrist (carpal)
19: Finger (digital
    or phalangeal)
20: Thigh (femoral)
21: Knee (genu)
22: Leg: (crural)
23: Foot (pedal)
24: Breast: (mammary)
25: Trunk: (torso, body
    without limbs)
26: Abdomen (abdominal)
27: Anterior surface of hand
    (palmar or volar)
28: Toes (digital)

LEGEND:

Axial

Appendicular

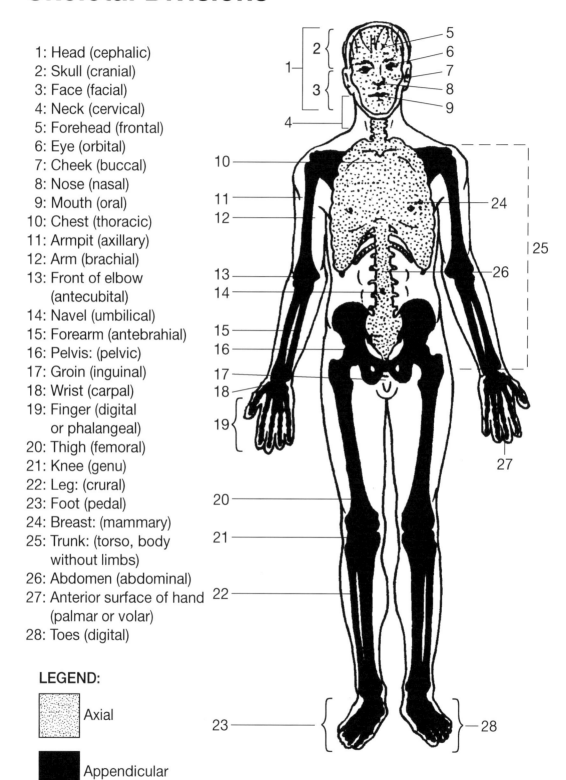

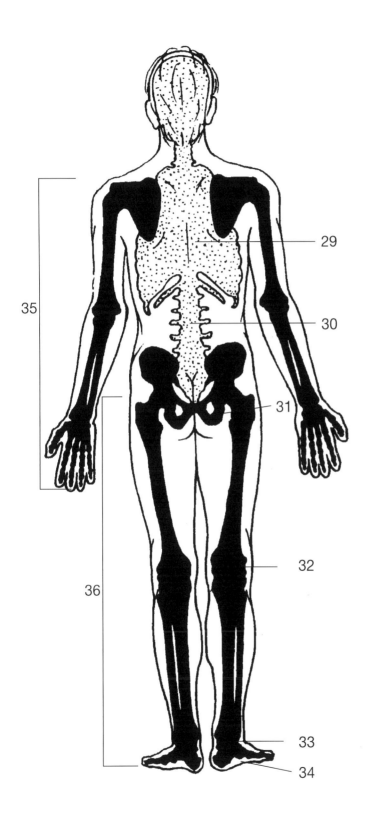

29: Back (dorsal)
30: Loin: (lumbar)
31: Buttock (gluteal)
32: Back of Knee: (popliteal)
33: Ankle (tarsal)
34: Sole of foot (plantar)

35: Upper Extremity
36: Lower Extremity

LEGEND:

 Axial

 Appendicular

Areas of the Abdomen

The abdomen is a large area of the lower trunk of the body. If a patient reported "abdominal pain", the physician or nurse would want to know more precisely where the pain was. In order to do this, the abdomen may be divided into smaller regions or areas:

Quadrants: A transverse plane and a midsagittal plane that cross at the umbilicus will divide the abdomen into four quadrants. Clinically, this is probably the division used more frequently. The pain of gallstones might then be described as the "right upper quadrant".

Nine areas: Two transverse planes and two sagittal planes divide the abdomen into nine areas.

Upper areas: Above the level of the rib cartilages are the left hypochondriac, epigastric, and right hypochondriac.

Middle areas: The left lumbar, umbilical and right lumbar.

Lower areas: Below the level of the top of the pelvic bone are the left iliac, hypogastric and right iliac. This division is often used in anatomical studies to describe the location of the organs. The liver, for example, is located in the epigastric and right hypochondriac areas.

The terms **anterior** and **posterior** are used to indicate the front and back of the body, respectively, so that when describing the relationship of two structures, they are said to be anterior or posterior.

In describing the hand, the terms **palmar** and **dorsal** surfaces are used in place of anterior and posterior; in describing the foot, the terms **plantar** and **dorsal** surfaces are used instead of lower and upper surfaces.

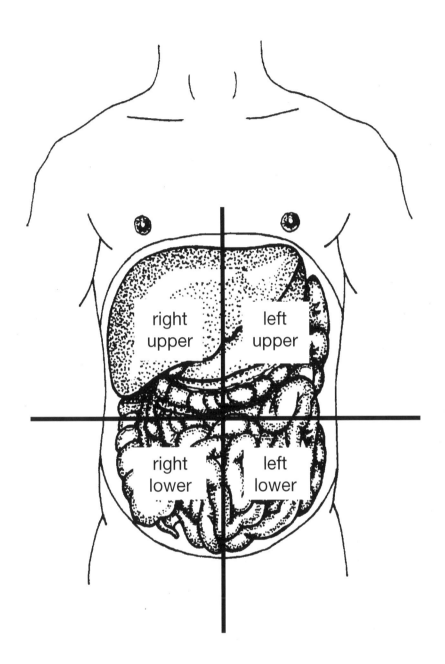

right
upper

left
upper

right
lower

left
lower

Division Of The Abdomen
Into Four Quadrants

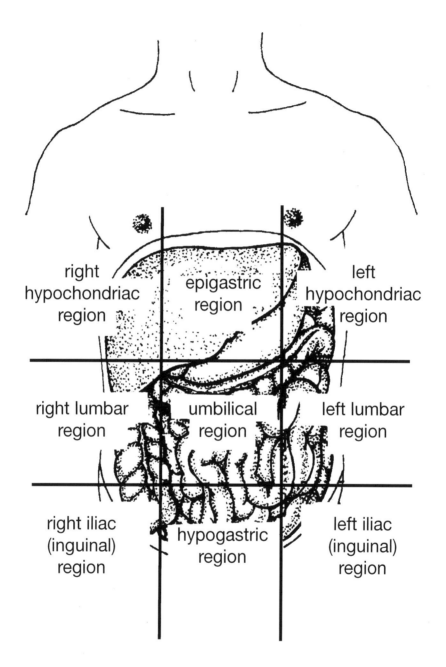

right
hypochondriac
region

epigastric
region

left
hypochondriac
region

right lumbar
region

umbilical
region

left lumbar
region

right iliac
(inguinal)
region

hypogastric
region

left iliac
(inguinal)
region

**The Nine Regions
Of The Abdomen**

The terms **proximal** and **distal** describe the relative distances from the roots of the limb; for example, the arm is proximal to the forearm and the hand is distal to the forearm.

Terms Related to Movement

The site where two or more bones come together is known as a **joint**. Some joints have no movement (sutures of skull), some have only slight movement and some are freely movable.

Flexion: Movement that takes place in a sagittal plane. For example, flexion of the elbow joint approximates the anterior surface of the forearm. It is usually an anterior movement, but it is occasionally posterior, as in the case of the knee joint.

Extension: Straightening of the joint; usually takes place in a posterior direction.

Lateral flexion: Movement of the trunk in the coronal plane.

Abduction: Movement of a limb away from the midline of the body in the coronal plane.

Adduction: Movement of a limb toward the body in the coronal plane. In the fingers and toes, abduction is applied to the spreading of these structures, and adduction is applied to the drawing together of these structures.

Rotation: Movement of a part of the body around its long axis. **Medial rotation** (internal rotation) is the movement that results in the anterior surface of the part facing medially; **lateral rotation** (external rotation) is the movement that results in the anterior surface of the part facing laterally.

Pronation of the forearm: Medial rotation of the forearm in such a manner that the palm of the hand faces posteriorly.

Supination of the forearm: Lateral rotation of the forearm from the pronated position, so that the palm of the hand comes to face anteriorly.

Circumduction: Combination in sequence of the movements of flexion, extension, abduction and adduction.

Protraction: To move forward.

Retraction: To move backward (used to described the forward and backward movement of the jaw at the temporomandibular joints).

Inversion: Movement of the foot so that the sole faces in a medial direction (supinated).

Eversion: Movement of the foot so that the sole faces in a lateral direction (pronated).

The Movements Of The Body

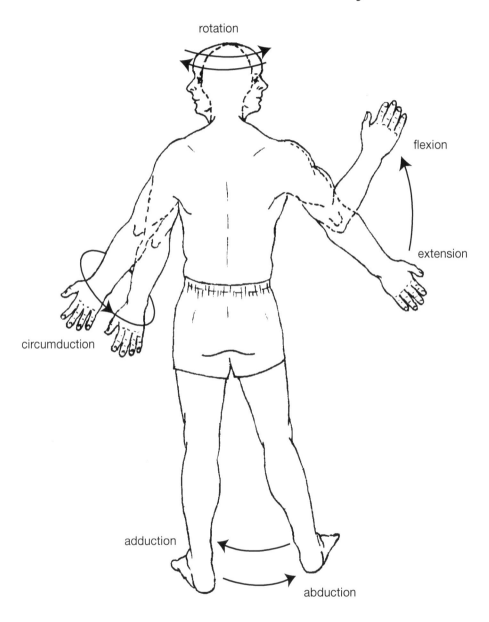

The Movements Of The Body
(continued)

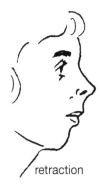

retraction

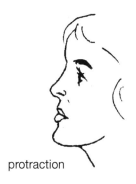

protraction

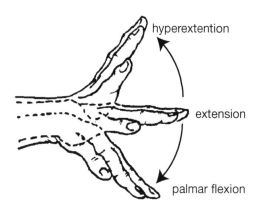

hyperextention

extension

palmar flexion

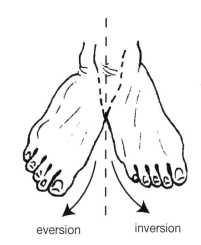

eversion   inversion

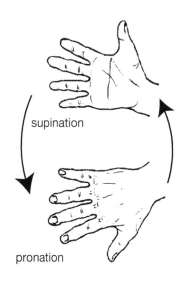

supination

pronation

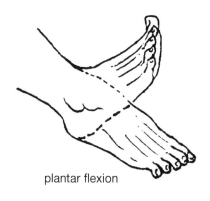

plantar flexion

CHAPTER 2
THE SKELETAL SYSTEM

Bones

Bones, the primary organs of the skeletal system, lie buried within the muscles and other soft tissues, providing a rigid framework and support structure of the whole body. Our skeleton (from the Greek word meaning "dried-up body") is a tower of bones arranged so that we can stand upright and balance ourselves. The skeleton is subdivided into two divisions: the **axial** skeleton, the bones that form the longitudinal axis of the body, and the **appendicular** skeleton, the bones of the limbs and girdles. In addition to the bones, ligaments and tendons bind the bones together at the joints. The joints give the body flexibility and allow movement to occur.

FUNCTIONS OF THE BONES

☞ SUPPORT: For the soft tissues of the body.
☞ MOVEMENT: Bones serve as levers and joints as fulcra.
☞ PROTECTION: To vital organs.
☞ STORAGE OF MINERALS: Calcium and phosphorus.
☞ BLOOD CELL FORMATION OR HAEMATOPOIESIS.

CLASSIFICATIONS OF BONES

The adult skeleton is composed of 206 bones (350 bones for infants). There are two basic types of **osseous**, or bone tissue: **compact** bone (cortical) is dense and looks smooth and homogeneous; **spongy** bone (cancellous) consists of a branching network of trabeculae. The trabeculae are arranged in such a manner as to resist the stresses and strains to which the bone is exposed. Bones come in many shapes and may be classified regionally or according to their general shape: **long, short, flat, irregular** and **sesamoid**.

• **Long bones**. These are found in the limbs (e.g. the humerus, the femur, the metacarpals, the metatarsals, and the phalanges); their length is greater than their width. They have a tubular shaft, the

diaphysis, and usually an **epiphysis** at each end. The part of the diaphysis that lies adjacent to the epiphyseal cartilage is called the **metaphysis**, which is the growth center that disappears at maturity, becoming vague epiphyseal lines. The shaft has a central **marrow cavity** (yellow marrow for adult and red marrow for infants; in adult bones, red marrow is confined to the cavities of spongy bone or flat bones and the epiphysis or some long bones).

The outer part of the shaft is composed of compact bone that is covered by a connective tissue sheath, the **periosteum**. The ends of the long bones are composed of spongy bone surrounded by a thin layer of compact bone. The articular surfaces of the ends of the bones are covered by **hyaline cartilage**.

• **Short bones.** These are found in the hand and foot (e.g. the scaphoid, lunate, talus and calcaneus) and are roughly cuboidal in shape. They are composed of cancellous bone (spongy) surrounded by a thin layer of compact bone. They are covered with periosteum and the articular surfaces are covered by hyaline cartilage.

• **Flat bones.** These are found in the vault of the skull (e.g. the frontal and parietal bones). They are composed of thin inner and outer layers of compact bone.

• **Irregular bones.** These include the vertebrae and the pelvic bones. They are composed of a thin shell of compact bone and an interior made up of cancellous bone.

• **Sesamoid bones.** These are small nodules of bone that are found in certain tendons where they rub over bony surfaces. The greater part of a sesamoid bone is buried in the tendon and the free surface is covered with cartilage. The largest sesamoid bone is the **patella**, which is located in the tendon of the **quadriceps femoris**. Other examples are found in the tendons of **flexor pollicis brevis** and **flexor hallucis brevis**. The function of a sesamoid bone is to reduce friction on the tendon; it may also alter the direction of a pull tendon.

Regional Classification of Bones

AXIAL SKELETON		# BONES

Skull:

	Cranium	8
	Face	14
	Auditory Ossicles	6

Trunk:

	Hyoid	1
	Verebrae	26
	Sternum	1
	Ribs	24

APPENDICULAR SKELETON

Shoulder Girdles:

	Clavical	2
	Scapula	2

Upper Extremities:

	Humerus	2
	Radius	2
	Ulna	2
	Carpals	16
	Metacarpals	10
	Phalanges	28

Pelvic Girdle:

	Innominate (hip) bone	2

Lower Extremities:

	Femur	2
	Patella	2
	Fibula	2
	Tibia	2
	Tarsals	14
	Metatarsals	10
	Phalanges	28
	TOTAL:	206

MICROSCOPIC ANATOMY OF COMPACT BONE

To the naked eye, spongy bone has a spiky, open appearance, whereas compact bone appears to be very dense. The needle-like threads of spongy bone that surround a network of spaces are called **trabeculae**. Compact or cortical bone does not contain a network of open spaces. Instead, the matrix is organized into numerous structural units called the **osteon** (haversian system). Each circular and tube-like osteon is composed of calcified matrix arranged in multiple layers resembling the rings of an onion. Each ring is called a **concentric lamella**. The circular rings or lamellae surround the **haversian canal**, which contains a blood vessel.

Bones are not lifeless structures. Within their hard, seemingly lifeless matrix are many living bone cells called **osteocytes**. Osteocytes lie between the hard layers of the lamellae in little spaces called **lacunae**. Note that tiny passageway or canals, called **canaliculi**, connect the lacunae with one another and with the central canal in each haversian system. Because of this elaborate network of canals, bone cells are well nourished in spite of the hardness of the matrix, and bone injuries heal quickly and well. The communication (and the haversian canals) is completed by **Volkmann's canals**, which run into the compact bone at right angles to the shaft.

DEVELOPMENT OF BONE

Bone is developed by two methods: **membranous** and **endocondral**. In the first method, the bone is developed directly from a connective tissue membrane; in the second, a cartilaginous model is first laid down and is later replaced by bone. The bones of the vault of the skull are developed rapidly by the membranous method in the embryo, and this serves to protect the underlying developing brain. At birth, small areas of membrane persist between the bones. This is important clinically since it allows the bones a certain amount of mobility, so that the skull can undergo molding during its descent through the female genital passages. At birth, ossification at the skull joints is not complete. Many of these bones are loosely joined by fibrous connective tissue or cartilage.

Six such joints, called **fontanelle**, occur at the angles of the parietal bone. The largest is the **anterior fontanelle** at the junction of the sagittal, coronal, and frontal sutures. The fontanelles, popularly referred to as "soft spots", permit the baby's head to be compressed slightly as it passes through the bony pelvis during birth. Apart from flat bones, which form on fibrous membranes, most bones develop using hyaline cartilage structures as their models. Most simply this process of bone formation, or ossification involves two major steps.

Osteoblasts are bone-building cells. They secrete the protein **collagen**, which forms the strong, elastic fibers of bone. A complex calcium phosphate called **apatite** is present in the tissue fluid. This compound automatically crystallizes around the collagen fibers, forming the hard matrix of bone. As the matrix forms around them, the osteoblasts become isolated within the small spaces called lacunae. The trapped osteoblasts are referred to as osteocytes.

Osteoclasts are the cells that break down bone, a process referred to as bone resorption. These bonebreaker cells move about secreting enzymes that digest bone. Osteoclasts and osteoblasts work side by side to shape bones and to form the precise grain needed in the finished bone.

The Internal Structure of a Long Bone

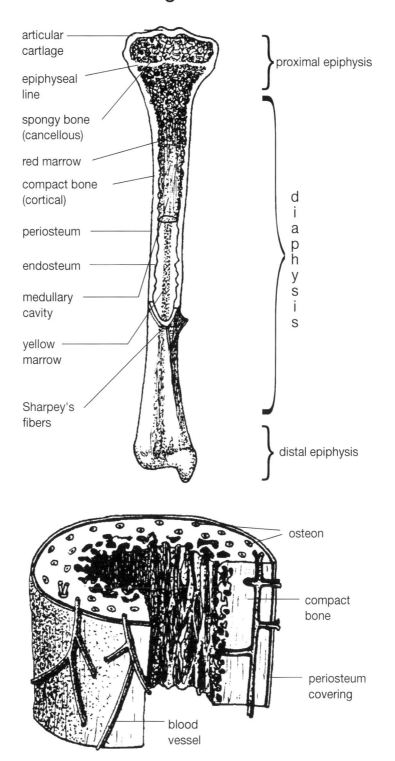

articular cartilage

epiphyseal line

spongy bone (cancellous)

red marrow

compact bone (cortical)

periosteum

endosteum

medullary cavity

yellow marrow

Sharpey's fibers

proximal epiphysis

d i a p h y s i s

distal epiphysis

osteon

compact bone

periosteum covering

blood vessel

The Internal Structure
of a Long Bone
(Continued)

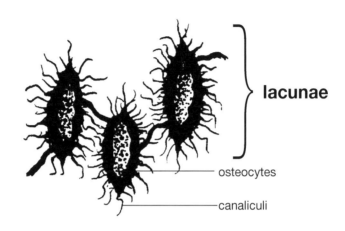

lacunae

osteocytes

canaliculi

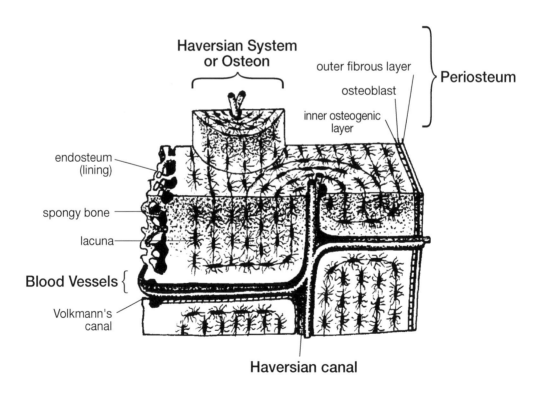

**Haversian System
or Osteon**

outer fibrous layer

osteoblast

inner osteogenic
layer

Periosteum

endosteum
(lining)

spongy bone

lacuna

Blood Vessels {

Volkmann's
canal

Haversian canal

Differences Between a Man's and a Woman's Skeleton

If you were to examine a male skeleton and a female skeleton placed side by side, you would probably notice first the difference in their sizes. Most male skeletons are larger than most female skeletons, a structural fact that seems to have no great functional importance.

The female pelvis is made so that the body of a baby can be cradled in it before birth and can pass through it during birth. Although the individual male hipbones (**os coxae**) are generally larger than the individual female hipbones, together the male hipbones form a narrower structure than do the female hipbones.

A man's pelvis is shaped something like a funnel, but a woman's pelvis has a broader, shallower shape, more like a basin. (Incidentally, the word pelvis means "basin"). Another difference is that the pelvic inlet or brim is normally much wider in the female than in the male. The angle at the front of the female pelvis where the two pubic bones join is wider than it is in the male.

Female Pelvis, Anterior View

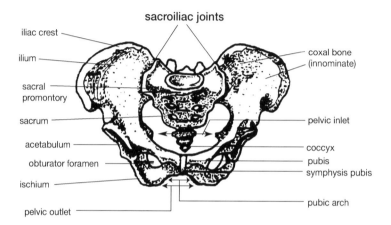

sacroiliac joints

iliac crest

ilium

sacral promontory

sacrum

acetabulum

obturator foramen

ischium

pelvic outlet

coxal bone (innominate)

pelvic inlet

coccyx

pubis

symphysis pubis

pubic arch

Male Pelvis, Anterior View

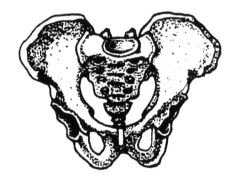

Cartilage

Cartilage is a form of connective tissue in which the cells and fibers are embedded in a gellike matrix, the latter being responsible for its firmness and resilience. Except on the exposed surfaces in joints, it is covered by a fibrous membrane called the **perichondrium**. There are three types of cartilage: **hyaline, fibrous**, and **elastic**.

☞ **Hyaline cartilage** has a high proportion of amorphous matrix that has the same refractive index as the fibers embedded in it. Throughout childhood and adolescence it plays an important part in the growth in length of long bones. Epiphyseal plates are composed of hyaline cartilage. It has a great resistance to wear and covers the articular surfaces of nearly all synovial joints. It is incapable of repair when fractured; the defect is filled with fibrous tissue.

☞ **Fibrocartilage** has a large number of collagen fibers embedded in a small amount of matrix. It is found in the discs within joints (e.g. the temporomandibular joint, sternoclavicular joints, knee joint) and on the articular surfaces of the clavicle and mandible. If damaged, it repairs itself slowly in a manner similar to fibrous tissue elsewhere. Joint discs have a poor blood supply and therefore do not repair themselves if damaged.

☞ **Elastic cartilage** possesses a large number of elastic fibers embedded in matrix. As would be expected, it is very flexible and is found in the auricle of the ear, the external auditory meatus, the auditory tube, and the epiglottis. If damaged, it repairs itself with fibrous tissue. Hyaline cartilage and fibrocartilage tend to calcify or even ossify later in life.

Joints (Articulations)

Every bone in the body, except one, connects to at least one other bone. In other words, every bone but one forms a joint with some other bone. The exception is the **hyoid bone** in the neck, to which the tongue anchors.

Joints may be classified into three types according to the degree of movement they allow: **synarthroses** (no movement), **amphiarthroses** (slight movement) and **diarthroses** (free movement). Differences in joint structure account for differences in the degree of movement that is possible.

☞ A **synarthroses** is a joint in which fibrous connective tissue grows between the articulating (joint) bones holding them close together. The joints between cranial bones are synarthroses, commonly called **sutures**.

☞ **Amphiarthroses** join bones to cartilage. The pubic symphysis of the pelvis and the intervertebral joints of the vertebral column are examples of amphiarthroses.

☞ Most of our joints by far are **diarthroses**, or **synovial** joints. Such joints allow considerable movement, sometimes in many directions and sometimes in only one or two directions. The ends of the bone forming a diarthrodial joint are covered with hyaline cartilage that lacks any sort of covering membrane. This articular cartilage also lacks nerves and blood vessels. The joint is surrounded by a connective tissue capsule called the **joint capsule**, made of tough fibrous connective tissue. This tissue is continuous with the periosteum of the bones but does not cover the articular cartilage. The joint capsule is lined with a smooth synovial membrane that secretes a lubricating **synovial fluid**. The joint capsule is generally reinforced with ligament, bands of fibrous connective tissue that connect the bones and also limit movement at the joint. Fluid filled sacs called

Joints

Hinge

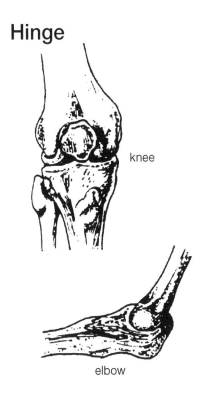

knee

elbow

Ball and Socket

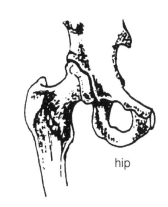

hip

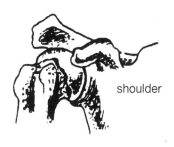

shoulder

Saddle

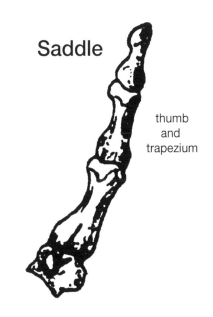

thumb
and
trapezium

Joints
(continued)

Condyloid

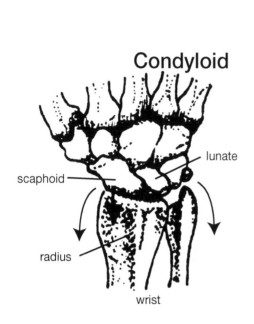

scaphoid

lunate

radius

wrist

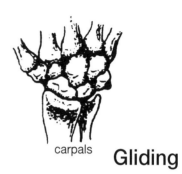

carpals

Gliding

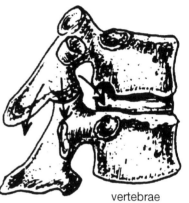

vertebrae

Pivot

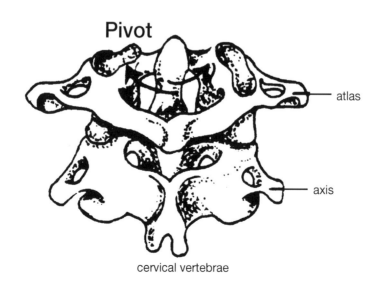

atlas

axis

cervical vertebrae

bursae are located between bone and tendons and between bone and some other tissues. Bursae cushion the movement of bone over other tissue. Inflammation of a bursa is a painful condition known as bursitis. There are six types of synovial joints: **gliding, condyloid, saddle, pivot, hinge,** and **ball and socket**.

The Skeletal System
Anterior View

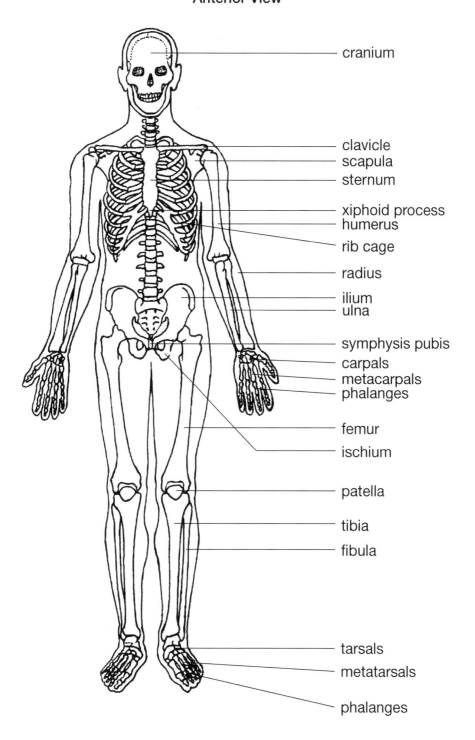

cranium

clavicle
scapula
sternum

xiphoid process
humerus
rib cage

radius

ilium
ulna

symphysis pubis
carpals
metacarpals
phalanges

femur
ischium

patella

tibia

fibula

tarsals

metatarsals

phalanges

The Skeletal System
Posterior View

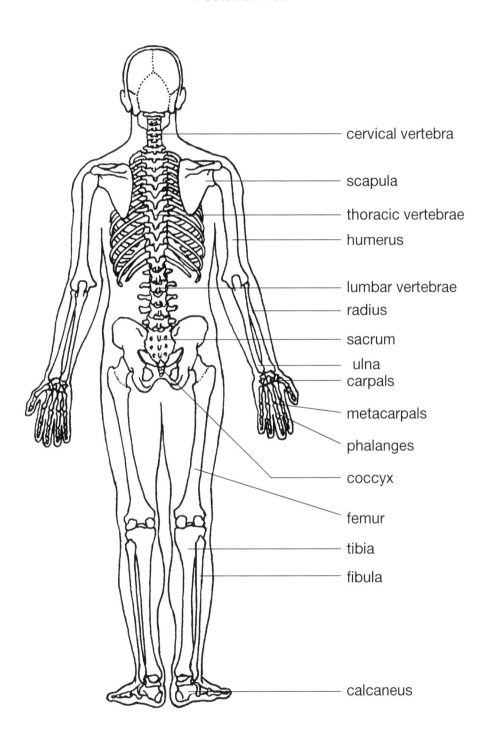

cervical vertebra

scapula

thoracic vertebrae

humerus

lumbar vertebrae

radius

sacrum

ulna

carpals

metacarpals

phalanges

coccyx

femur

tibia

fibula

calcaneus

The Skull
Anterior View

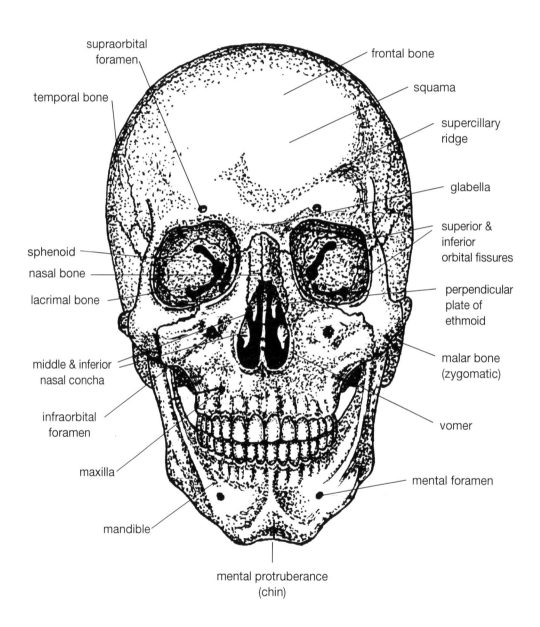

supraorbital foramen

temporal bone

frontal bone

squama

supercillary ridge

glabella

sphenoid

nasal bone

lacrimal bone

superior & inferior orbital fissures

perpendicular plate of ethmoid

middle & inferior nasal concha

malar bone (zygomatic)

infraorbital foramen

vomer

maxilla

mandible

mental foramen

mental protruberance (chin)

The Skull
Lateral View

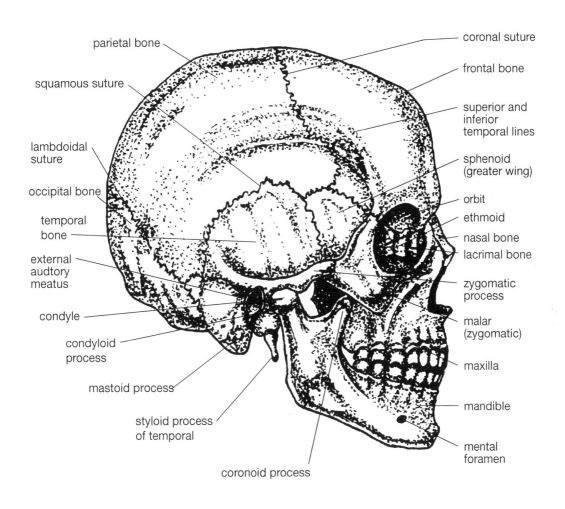

parietal bone

squamous suture

lambdoidal suture

occipital bone

temporal bone

external audtory meatus

condyle

condyloid process

mastoid process

styloid process of temporal

coronoid process

coronal suture

frontal bone

superior and inferior temporal lines

sphenoid (greater wing)

orbit

ethmoid

nasal bone

lacrimal bone

zygomatic process

malar (zygomatic)

maxilla

mandible

mental foramen

The Skull
Posterior View

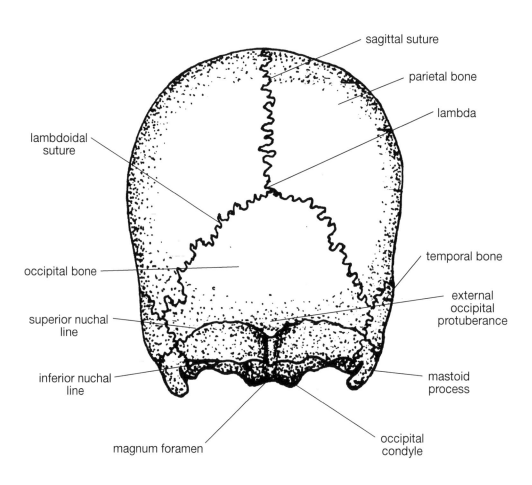

sagittal suture

parietal bone

lambda

lambdoidal
suture

temporal bone

external
occipital
protuberance

occipital bone

superior nuchal
line

inferior nuchal
line

mastoid
process

magnum foramen

occipital
condyle

Right Pelvis
lateral View

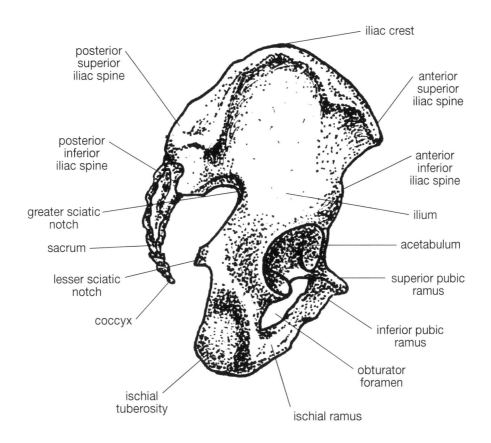

iliac crest

posterior superior iliac spine

anterior superior iliac spine

posterior inferior iliac spine

anterior inferior iliac spine

greater sciatic notch

ilium

sacrum

acetabulum

lesser sciatic notch

superior pubic ramus

coccyx

inferior pubic ramus

obturator foramen

ischial tuberosity

ischial ramus

Vertebral Column

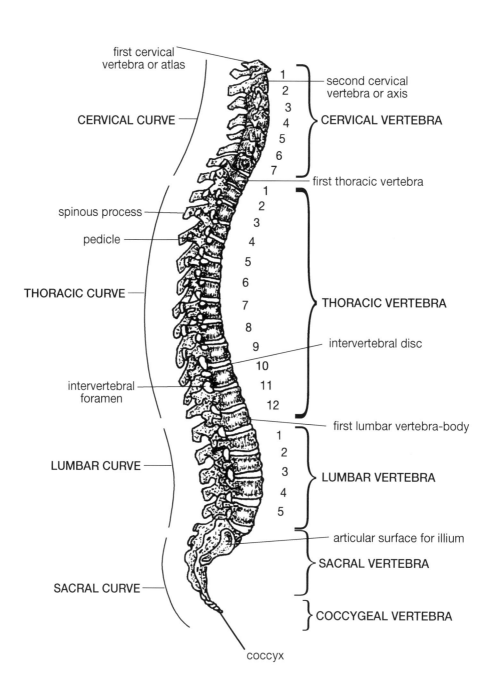

first cervical vertebra or atlas

second cervical vertebra or axis

CERVICAL CURVE

CERVICAL VERTEBRA

1
2
3
4
5
6
7

first thoracic vertebra

spinous process

pedicle

1
2
3
4
5
6
7
8
9
10
11
12

THORACIC CURVE

THORACIC VERTEBRA

intervertebral disc

intervertebral foramen

first lumbar vertebra-body

1
2
3
4
5

LUMBAR CURVE

LUMBAR VERTEBRA

articular surface for illium

SACRAL VERTEBRA

SACRAL CURVE

COCCYGEAL VERTEBRA

coccyx

Right Humerus

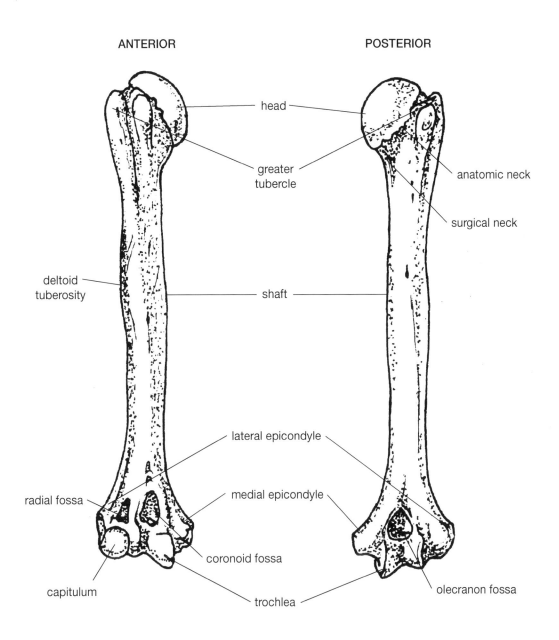

ANTERIOR

POSTERIOR

head

greater
tubercle

anatomic neck

surgical neck

deltoid
tuberosity

shaft

lateral epicondyle

radial fossa

medial epicondyle

coronoid fossa

capitulum

trochlea

olecranon fossa

Right Radius and Ulna

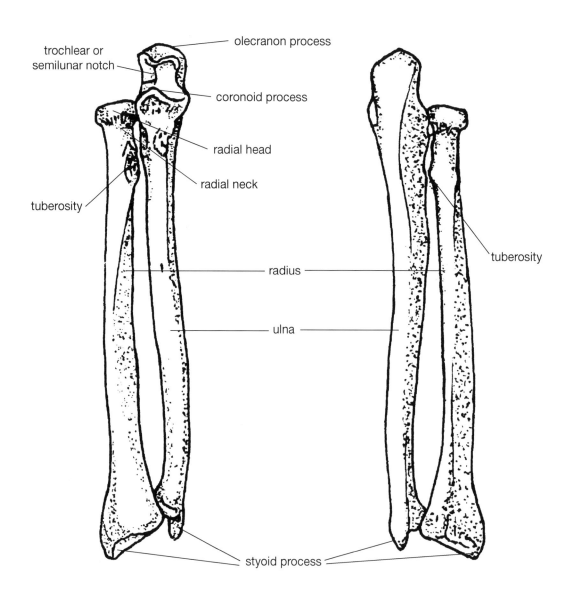

trochlear or
semilunar notch

olecranon process

coronoid process

radial head

radial neck

tuberosity

tuberosity

radius

ulna

styoid process

Right Femur

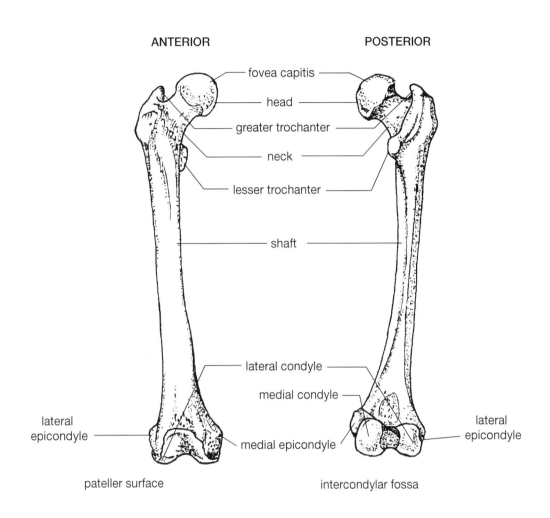

ANTERIOR

POSTERIOR

fovea capitis

head

greater trochanter

neck

lesser trochanter

shaft

lateral condyle

medial condyle

lateral
epicondyle

lateral
epicondyle

medial epicondyle

pateller surface

intercondylar fossa

Right Patella

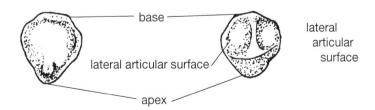

base

lateral
articular
surface

lateral articular surface

apex

Right Tibia / Fibula

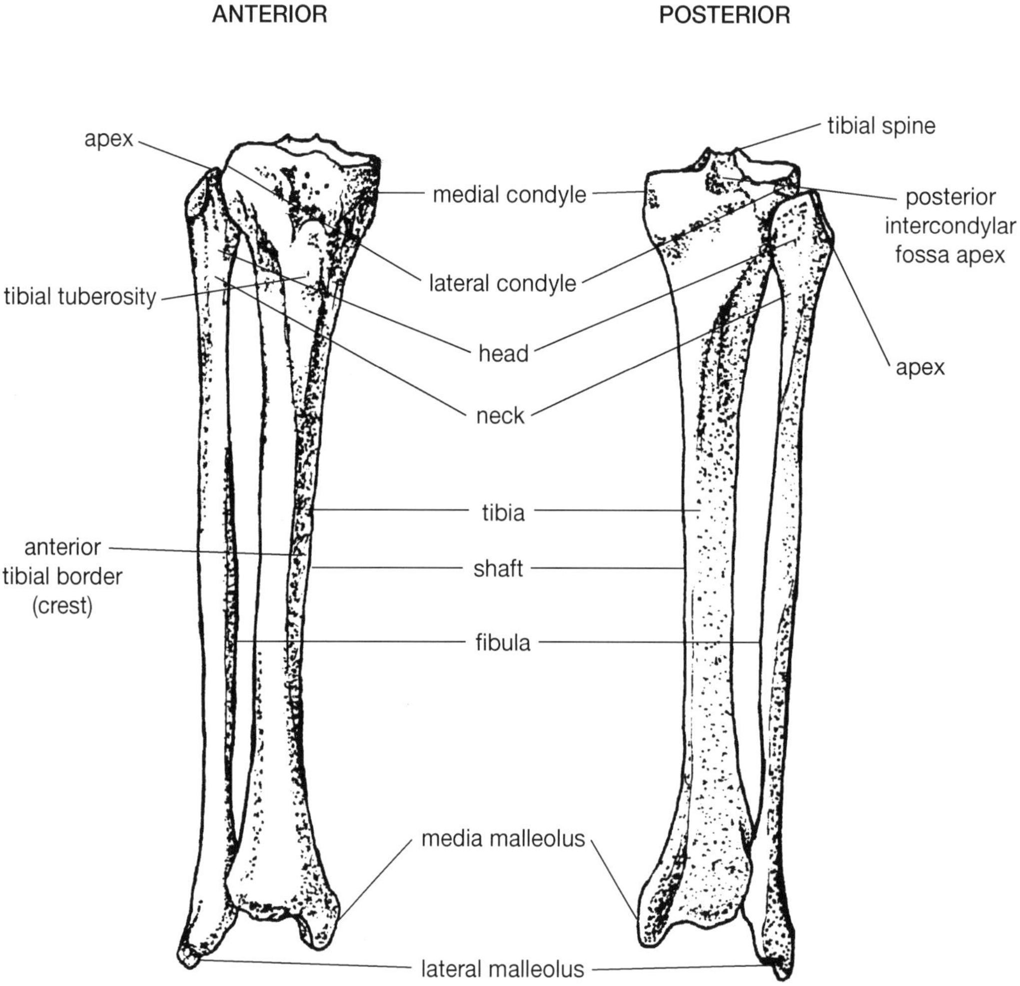

ANTERIOR

POSTERIOR

apex

medial condyle

tibial spine

posterior
intercondylar
fossa apex

tibial tuberosity

lateral condyle

head

neck

apex

tibia

anterior
tibial border
(crest)

shaft

fibula

media malleolus

lateral malleolus

Right Foot

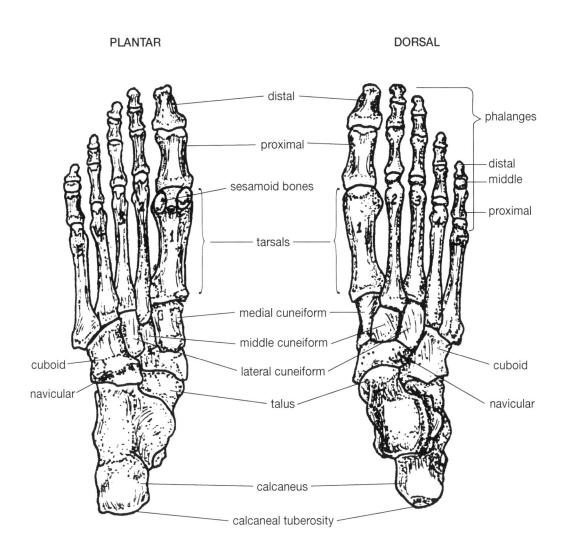

PLANTAR

DORSAL

distal

proximal

sesamoid bones

tarsals

medial cuneiform

middle cuneiform

cuboid

navicular

lateral cuneiform

talus

calcaneus

calcaneal tuberosity

phalanges

distal
middle

proximal

cuboid

navicular

Right Foot
(Dorsal Aspect)

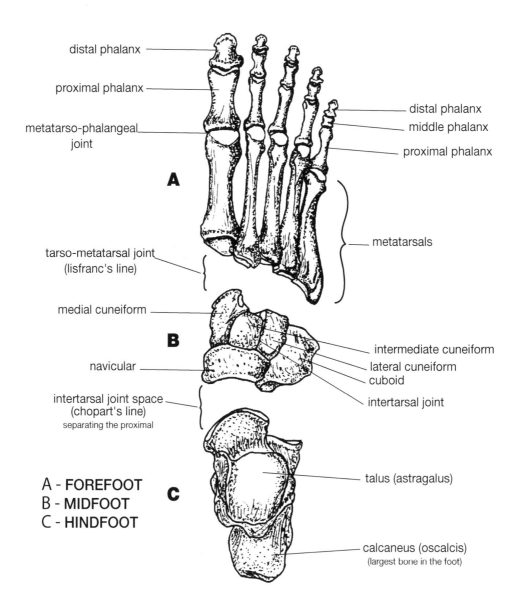

distal phalanx

proximal phalanx

metatarso-phalangeal joint

distal phalanx

middle phalanx

proximal phalanx

A

metatarsals

tarso-metatarsal joint (lisfranc's line)

medial cuneiform

B

intermediate cuneiform

lateral cuneiform

cuboid

navicular

intertarsal joint

intertarsal joint space (chopart's line)
separating the proximal

talus (astragalus)

A - **FOREFOOT**
B - **MIDFOOT**
C - **HINDFOOT**

C

calcaneus (oscalcis)
(largest bone in the foot)

Anterior View of Hand

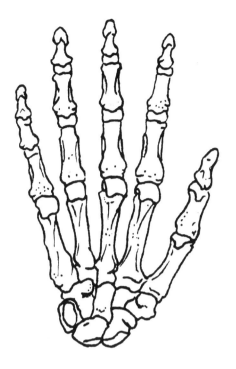

Posterior View of Hand

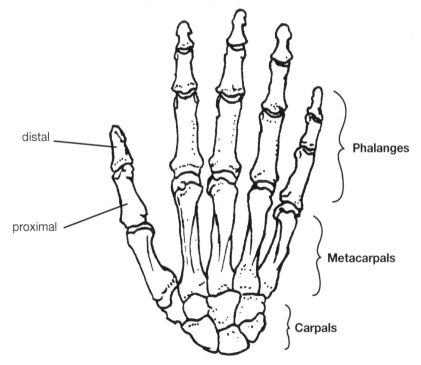

distal

proximal

Phalanges

Metacarpals

Carpals

Right Hand
Anterior View
(Volar or Palmar Aspect)

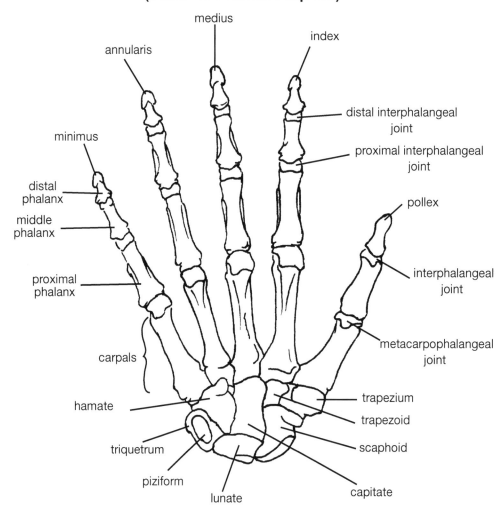

medius

index

annularis

distal interphalangeal joint

proximal interphalangeal joint

minimus

distal phalanx

middle phalanx

pollex

interphalangeal joint

proximal phalanx

carpals

metacarpophalangeal joint

hamate

trapezium

trapezoid

triquetrum

scaphoid

piziform

capitate

lunate

Eight Carpal Bones from Lateral to Medial, Proximal to Distal

Sally	*Left*	*The*	*Party*
Scaphoid (Navicular)	Lunate (Semi-lunar)	Triquetrum (Pyramidal)	Pisiform (Lentiform)
To	*Take*	*Carlos*	*Home*
Trapezium (Greater Multangular)	Trapezoid (Lesser Multangular)	Capitate (Os Magnum)	Hamate (Hook-like)

CHAPTER 3
THE MUSCULAR SYSTEM

The Muscular System

This chapter is devoted to muscle, which contributes 40% to 45% of body weight. Running, speaking, chewing, circulating blood, and moving food along the digestive tract are all body movements dependant on the actions of muscles. The three types of muscles are **smooth** (visceral), **cardiac**, and **skeletal** (striated) muscle. Of the three types, cardiac muscle is the toughest. The cardiac muscle (heart) has seen thousands of people through lives of more than 100 years. In such cases, the heart will have beaten 4 billion times and pumped 600,000 tons of blood. In this chapter we will focus on skeletal muscle, the voluntary muscles that attach to bone.

MUSCLE STRUCTURE

Muscle tissue consists of specialized contractile cells or **muscle fibers** that are grouped together and arranged in a highly organized way. A covering of connective tissue called the **epimysium** surrounds the skeletal muscle. Muscle fibers are arranged in bundles known as **fascicles**. Each fascicle is wrapped by connective tissue called **perimysium**. Finally, individual muscle fibers are surrounded by a connective tissue covering called endomysium. The epimysium, perimysium, and **endomysium** are continuous. Extensions of epimysium form **tendons**, tough cords of connective tissue that anchor muscle to bone. Each muscle fiber is a spindleshaped cell with many nuclei. The cell membrane, known in a muscle cell as the **sarcolemma**, has multiple inward extensions that form a set of **T-tubules** (transverse tubules). The cytoplasm of a muscle fiber is referred to as **sarcoplasm**, and the endoplasmic reticulum as **sarcoplasmic reticulum**.

Threadlike structures called **myofibrils** run lengthwise through the muscle fiber. The myofibrils are composed of two types of even tinier structures called **myofilaments**. The thick myofilaments, called **myosin** filaments, consist mainly of the protein myosin, whereas the thin **actin** filaments consist of the protein actin. Myosin and actin filaments are arranged lengthwise in the muscle fibers so that they overlap. Their overlapping produces a pattern of bands, or striations, characteristic of striated muscle. A **sarcomere** is a unit of thick and thin filaments. Sarcomeres are joined at their ends by an interweaving of filaments called the **z-line**.

MUSCLE CONTRACTION

Muscle cells have some special functional properties that enable them to perform their duties. The first of these is **irritability**, the ability to receive and respond to a stimulus. The second, **contractibility**, is the ability to shorten (forcibly) when an adequate stimulus is received. Skeletal muscle must be stimulated by nerve impulses to contract. One **motor neuron** (nerve cell) may stimulate a few muscle cells or hundreds of them, depending on the particular muscle and the work it does.

One neuron and all the skeletal muscles it stimulates is a **motor unit**. When a long threadlike extension of the neuron, called the **nerve fiber** or **axon**, reaches the muscle, it branches into a number of axonal terminals, each of which forms a junction with the sarcolemma of a different muscle cell. These junctions are called **neuromuscular** junctions. Although the nerve endings and the muscle cell membranes are very close, they never touch. The gap between them, the **synaptic cleft**, is filled with tissue (interstitial) fluid.

Now that we have described the structure of the neuromuscular junction, we are ready to examine what happens there. When the nerve impulse reaches the axonal terminals, a chemical referred to as a **neurotransmitter** is released. The specific neurotransmitter that stimulates skeletal muscle cells is **acetylcholine**, or **ACH**. The acetylcholine diffuses across the **myoneural** (muscle nerve) junction between the neuron and the muscle cell and combines with receptors on the surface of the muscle cell. This initiates an impulse (an electrical current) that spreads over the sarcolemma. The electrical current generated is known as **action potential**.

Muscle Structure

Microscopic Structure
Of The Skin

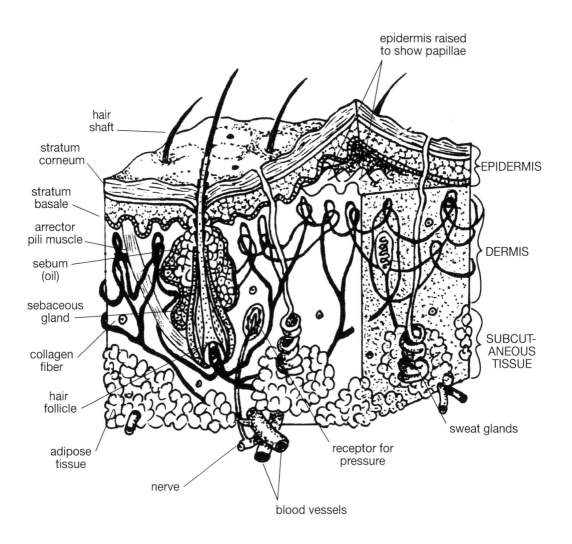

epidermis raised
to show papillae

hair
shaft

stratum
corneum

stratum
basale

arrector
pili muscle

sebum
(oil)

sebaceous
gland

collagen
fiber

hair
follicle

adipose
tissue

nerve

blood vessels

receptor for
pressure

sweat glands

EPIDERMIS

DERMIS

SUBCUT-
ANEOUS
TISSUE

Muscle Structure
(continued)

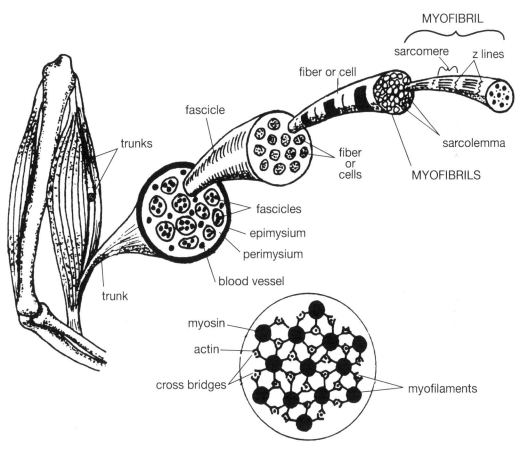

MYOFIBRIL

sarcomere

z lines

fiber or cell

sarcolemma

MYOFIBRILS

fascicle

trunks

fiber
or
cells

fascicles

epimysium

perimysium

blood vessel

trunk

myosin

actin

cross bridges

myofilaments

Cross Section Of A Myofibril

Excessive acetylcholine is broken down by the enzyme **cholinesterase**. The impulse spreads through the **T-tubules** and stimulates the sarcoplasmic reticulum to release calcium ions into the sarcoplasm. The calcium induces a process that uncovers binding sites on the actin filaments, cross bridges along the myosin filaments attached to the exposed binding sites on the actin filaments. This process is powered by energy from **ATP (adenosine triphosphate)** molecules. Cross bridges flex and attach to new binding sites. As this process continues, the actin filaments slide past the myosin filaments, shortening the muscle.

Functions of Skeletal Muscle

The three primary functions of the musculature system are:
☞ Movement
☞ Posture or muscle tone
☞ Heat production

MOVEMENT

Muscles move bones by **pulling** on them. Because the length of a skeletal muscle becomes shorter as its fibers contract, the bone to which the muscle attaches moves closer together. As a rule, only the insertion bone moves. The origin bone stays put, holding firm, while the insertion bone moves toward it. One tremendously important function of skeletal muscle contractions, therefore, is to produce body movement. A simple rule will help you understand muscle actions: **A muscle's insertion bone moves towards its origin bone.**

Voluntary muscular movements are normally smooth and free of jerks and tremors because skeletal muscles generally work in coordinated teams, not singly. Several muscles contract while others relax to produce almost any movement that you can imagine. Of all the muscles contracting simultaneously, the one that is mainly responsible for producing a particular movement is called the **prime mover** for that movement, while the other muscles that help in producing the movement are called **synergists**. As prime movers and synergists contract muscles, other muscles called **antagonists** relax. When the antagonist muscles contract, they produce a movement opposite to that of the prime movers and their synergist muscles.

POSTURE

We are able to maintain our body position because of a specialized type of skeletal muscle contraction called **tonic (tone) contraction**. In a tonic contraction, relatively few muscle fibers shorten at one time; the muscle as a whole does not shorten, and no movement occurs. Consequently, tonic contractions do not move any body parts; however, they do hold muscles in position. In other words, muscle tone maintains **posture**. Skeletal muscle tone maintains posture by counteracting the pull of gravity. Gravity tends to pull the head and trunk down and forward, but the tone in certain back and neck muscles pulls just hard enough in the opposite direction to overcome the force of gravity and hold the head and trunk erect.

HEAT PRODUCTION

Healthy survival depends on our ability to maintain a constant body temperature. A fever or elevation in body temperature of only a degree or two above 37° C (98.6° F) is always a sign of illness. Just as serious is a drop in body temperature. Any decrease below normal – a condition called **hypothermia** – drastically affects cellular activity and normal body function. Most of the heat required to produce a muscle contraction is obtained from the ATP molecules. Most of the energy released during the breakdown of the ATP during a muscular contraction is used to shorten the muscle fiber; however, some of the energy is lost as heat during the reaction. This heat helps to maintain our body temperature at a constant level.

FATIGUE

If muscle cells are stimulated repeatedly without adequate periods of rest, the strength of the muscle contraction decreases, resulting in **fatigue**. If repeated stimulation occurs, the strength of the contraction continues to decrease, and eventually the muscle loses its ability to contract.

During exercise, the stored ATP required for muscle contraction becomes depleted. Formation of more ATP results in a rapid consumption of oxygen and nutrients, often outstripping the ability of the muscle's blood supply to replenish them. When oxygen supplies run low, the muscle cells switch to a type of energy conversion that does not require oxygen. This process produces **lactic acid** that may result in muscle soreness after exercise. The term **oxygen debt** describes the continued increased metabolism that must occur in a cell to remove excess lactic acid and replace depleted energy reserves. Labored breathing after cessation of exercise is required for the metabolic effect. In a good example of **homeostasis** at work, the body returns the cell's energy and oxygen reserves to normal resting levels.

TETANUS

Nerve impulses are generally delivered to a muscle at a rapid rate. With such rapidly repeated stimulation, the muscle contracts repeatedly without relaxing between each contraction. The individual contractions fuse into a single, smooth, sustained contraction. This type of muscle response is referred to as **tetanus**. (This type of tetanus is normal and has nothing to do with the disorder tetanus that causes muscles to go into uncontrollable spasms).

ISOTONIC AND ISOMETRIC CONTRACTION

When you lift a heavy object or bend your elbow, muscles shorten and thicken as they contract. Muscle tone remains the same. We usually think of muscle contraction in terms of this type of **isotonic contraction**. However, if you push against a table or wall, no movement results. Muscle length does not appreciably change but muscle tension may increase greatly. This type of muscle contraction is referred to as **isometric contraction**.

ORIGIN, INSERTION AND ACTION

Skeletal muscles produce movements, or **actions**, by pulling on tendons, which in turn pull on bones. Most muscles pass across a joint and are attached to the bones that form a joint. When the muscle contracts it draws one bone toward or away from the bone with which it articulates (forms a joint). The attachment of the muscle to the less movable bone is called its **origin**. The attachment of the muscle to the more movable bone is its **insertion**.

Specific Muscles and Their Actions

BICEPS FEMORIS
Origin: SHORT HEAD: Lateral lip of linea aspera, supracondylar ridge, lateral intermuscular septum; LONG HEAD: Ischial tuberosity, sacrotuberous ligament
Insertion: Head of fibula, lateral condyle of tibia
Action: Extension and adduction of thigh, flexion of leg

BRACHIALIS
O: Anterolateral and anteriomedial surface of humerus, medial and lateral intermuscular septum
I: Ulnar tuberosity, coronoid tuberosity
A: Flexion of forearm, flexion of arm against resistance

BRACHIORADIALIS
O: Upper 2/3 of lateral epicondylar ridge of humerus, lateral intermuscular septum
I: Lateral side of base of styloid process of radius
A: Flexion of forearm, supination when arm is extended and pronated, pronation when arm is fixed and supinated

CORACOBRACHIALIS
O: Coracoid process of scapula, tendon of caput breve of biceps
I: Medial surface and ridge of proximal humeral shaft
A: Adduction and flexion in shoulder

DELTOID
O: Lateral 1/3 of clavicle, acromion, and spine of scapula
I: Deltoid tuberosity of humerus

A: Abduction, flexion, and extension of arm; internal and external rotation

GASTROCNEMIUS
O: MEDIAL HEAD: Medial condyle of femur, femoral margin of capsule of knee joint, small area of back of femur; LATERAL HEAD: Lateral condyle of femur, small area behind lateral condyle
I: A common tendon with tibial soleus muscle (calcaneal tendon)
A: Plantar flexion and supination of foot, flexion of knee, raising of heel

GLUTEUS MAXIMUS
O: Lateral portions of lower sacral and coccygeal vertebrae, back of sacrotuberous ligament, outer lip of iliac crest, and outer surface of ilium, thoracolumbar fascia
I: Gluteal tuberosity of femur, iliotibial tract
A: Extension and external rotation of thigh, tension of fascia lata and iliotibial band, keeps extended knee joint steady

GLUTEUS MEDIUS
O: Ventral 3/4 of iliac crest, outer surface of ilium between anterior and posterior gluteal lines
I: External surface of greater trochanter, oblique ridge on lateral surface of greater trochanter
A: Abduction and extension of thigh, external rotation (posterior part) internal rotation (anterior part)

GLUTEUS MINIMUS
O: Outer surface of ilium between anterior and inferior gluteal lines, margin of greater sciatic notch; capsule of hip joint
I: Anterior border of greater trochanter
A: Abduction of thigh, internal rotation (anterior part); flexion (anterior part) and extension (posterior part) of thigh

GRACILIS
O: Inferior half of symphysis pubis, superior half of pubic arch
I: Upper part of medial surface of tibia
A: Adduction, flexion of thigh, external rotation of thigh

ILIACUS

O: Greater part of iliac fossa, iliac crest, iliolumbar ligament, and anterior sacroiliac ligaments

I: Femur immediately distal to lesser trochanter

A: Flexion and external rotation of thigh at hip joint with flexed leg, tilting forward of pelvis

ILEOPSOAS

Composed of **medial iliacus** and **medial psoas**

INFRASPINATUS

O: Vertebral 3/4 of infraspinatus fossa, lower surface of scapular spine

I: Middle facet of greater tubercle of humerus

A: External rotation of arm; UPPER PART: abduction of arm; LOWER PART: adduction of arm

LATISSIMUS DORSI

O: Thoracolumbar fascia, spinous and infraspinous ligaments T6-L3, crest of ilium, last three or four ribs

I: Crest of lesser tubercle of humerus, intertubercular groove

A: Adduction and internal rotation of arm

PECTORALIS MAJOR

O: CLAVICULAR PART: Anterior aspect of clavicle; STERNOCOSTAL PART: Side and front of sternum, front of cartilage of ribs 2 – 6; ABDOMINAL PART: Aponeurosis of external oblique muscle

I: Greater tubercle of humerus

A: Flexion and adduction of arm, internal rotation of arm, raising of ribs in forced inspiration

PECTORALIS MINOR

O: Aponeurotic slips from ribs 2-5

I: Medial border, upper surface of coracoid process of scapula

A: Pulling forward of scapula, pulling downward of lateral angle of scapula, aids in raising ribs

PERONEUS BREVIS
O: Lateral surface of fibula, intermuscular septa
I: Dorsal aspect of tuberosity of metatarsal 5
A: Eversion of foot (plantar flexion of foot)

PERONEUS LONGUS
O: Head of upper 2/3 of lateral surface of fibula, intermuscular septa
I: Base of metatarsal 1, lateral side of cuneiform 1
A: Dorsiflexion and abduction of foot, eversion of foot

PERONEUS TERTIUS
O: Lower part of fibula, intermuscular septa
I: Metatarsal 5
A: Eversion and plantar flexion of foot

PLANTARIS
O: Distal part of lateral line of linea aspera
I: Achilles tendon
A: Raising of heel, flexion of leg at knee joint

POPLITEUS
O: Lateral aspect of lateral condyle of femur
I: Popliteal line of tibia, surface of shaft of tibia
A: Internal rotation of leg, flexion of leg

PRONATOR QUADRATUS
O: Ventral surface of distal 1/4 of ulna
I: Ventral surface of radius, triangular area above ulnar notch
A: Pronation of forearm

PRONATOR TERES
O:HUMERAL HEAD: Central surface of medial epicondyle, overlying fascia and intermuscular septa; ULNAR HEAD: Medial border of coronoid process
I: Ventral surface of radius
A: Pronation and flexion of forearm

PSOAS MAJOR
O: Intervertebral discs of lowest thoracic and all lumbar vertebrae, bodies of lumbar vertebrae, transverse processes of lumbar vertebrae
I: Lesser trochanter
A: Tilting of thigh at hip joint, rotation of thigh, flexion of spine and pelvis, abduction of lumbar part of spine

PSOAS MINOR
O: Lowest thoracic and first lumbar vertebrae, intervertebral discs between these vertebrae
I: Iliac fascia, iliopubic eminence
A: Tilting forward of pelvis, tenses iliac fascia

RECTUS FEMORIS
O: LONG HEAD: Anterior inferior spine of ilium; SHORT HEAD: Posterosuperior surface of rim of acetabulum
I: Proximal border of the patella, tuberosity of tibia
A: Flexion of thigh at the hip joint, extension of leg

SEMIMEMBRANOSUS
O: Ischial tuberosity
I: Back of medial condyle of tibia, lateral condyle of femur, capsule of knee joint
A: Internal rotation and flexion of leg, extension and adduction of thigh, internal rotation of thigh

SEMITENDINOSUS
O: Medidorsal facet of tuberosity of ischium
I: Proximal part of medial surface of tibia
A: Extension and adduction of thigh, internal rotation of thigh, flexion of leg, internal rotation of leg (knee flexed)

SOLEUS
O: Head and posterior surface of fibula, popliteal line and middle 1/3 of tibia, intermuscular septum
I: A common tendon with gastrocnemius muscle (calcaneal tendon)
A: Plantar flexion of foot at ankle joint, raising of heel

SUBSCAPULARIS
O: Costal surface of scapula, intermuscular septa between it and the teres muscles

I: Lesser tubercle and shaft of humerus

A: Internal rotation of humerus, adduction of humerus, fixation of head of humerus

SUPINATOR
O: Lateral epicondyle of humerus, radial collateral ligament of elbow joint, small crista of ulna

I: Upper part of radius between anterior and posterior oblique lines

A: Supination of forearm

SUPRASPINATUS
O: Medial 2/3 of supraspinous fossa, medial part of enveloping fascia

I: Superior facet of greater tubercle of humerus

A: Abduction of arm, fixation of head of humerus during abduction

TENSOR FASCIAE LATAE
O: External lip of iliac crest, fascia lata

I: Iliotibial band

A: Flexion, internal rotation and abduction of thigh; flexion, abduction and external rotation of pelvis; external rotation of tibia

TERES MAJOR
O: Dorsal surface of inferior angle of scapula, intermuscular septum

I: Crest of lesser tubercle of humerus

A: Adduction of arm, medial rotation of arm, extension of arm

TERES MINOR
O: Axillary border of infraspinous fossa, fascia infraspinata, intermuscular septum

I: Inferior facet of greater tubercle of humerus

A: Lateral rotation of arm, adduction

TIBIALIS ANTERIOR
O: Distal part of lateral condyle of tibia, lateral surface of proximal 1/2 of tibia, interosseous membrane and intermuscular septum

I: Medial surface of cuneiform 1, base of metatarsal 1

A: Dorsiflexion of foot at ankle, inversion of foot (foot dorsiflexed)

TIBIALIS POSTERIOR
O: Middle 1/3 of posterior surface of tibia, lateral 1/2 of popliteal line, part of body of fibula, interosseous membrane and intermuscular septa

I: Tubercle of navicular bone and cuneiform 1, cuneiform 4, and base of metatarsal 4, sulcus of cuboid, capsule of naviculocuneiform joint

A: Inversion of foot, support of foot arches (plantarflexion of foot)

TRAPEZIUS
O: Superior nuchal line, external protuberance of occipital bone, nuchal ligament, supraspinous ligament from 7th cervical to 12th thoracic vertebrae

I: Lateral third of clavicle, acromion and upper border of spine of scapula, medial end of spine of scapula

A: Draws scapula towards spine, exorotation of scapula, draws shoulder upward, extension of head and bending of neck

TRICEPS BRACHII
O: LONG HEAD: Infraglenoid tuberosity of scapula; LATERAL HEAD: Posterior surface of humerus, lateral intermuscular septum; MEDIAL HEAD: Posterior surface of humerus below radial groove, medial and lateral intermuscular septa

I: Olecranon, dorsal fascia of forearm

A: Extension of elbow joint, adduction of arm (long head), maintenance of elbow in extended position

VASTUS INTERMEDIUS
O: Anterolateral surface of shaft of femur, distal 1/2 of lateral margin of linea aspera

I: Aponeurosis of insertion of vastus lateralis proximal margin of patella

A: Extension of knee

VASTUS LATERALIS

O: Anterior inferior margin of greater trochanter, lateral intermuscular septum

I: Proximal border of patella, front of lateral condyle of tibia

A: Extension of knee

VASTUS MEDIALIS

O: Linea aspera and distal 1/2 of intertrochanteric line

I: Medial and proximal margin of patella

A: Extension of knee

The Muscular System
(Anterior View)

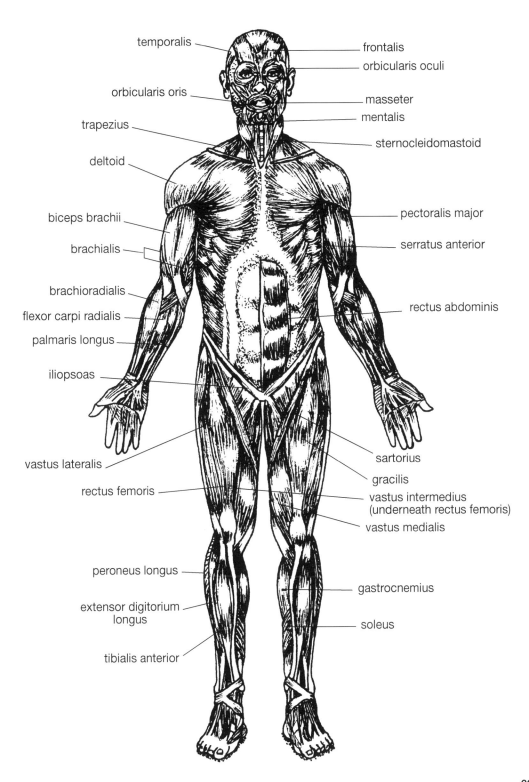

temporalis

frontalis

orbicularis oculi

orbicularis oris

masseter

mentalis

trapezius

sternocleidomastoid

deltoid

biceps brachii

pectoralis major

brachialis

serratus anterior

brachioradialis

flexor carpi radialis

rectus abdominis

palmaris longus

iliopsoas

vastus lateralis

sartorius

rectus femoris

gracilis

vastus intermedius
(underneath rectus femoris)

vastus medialis

peroneus longus

gastrocnemius

extensor digitorium
longus

soleus

tibialis anterior

The Muscular System
(Posterior View)

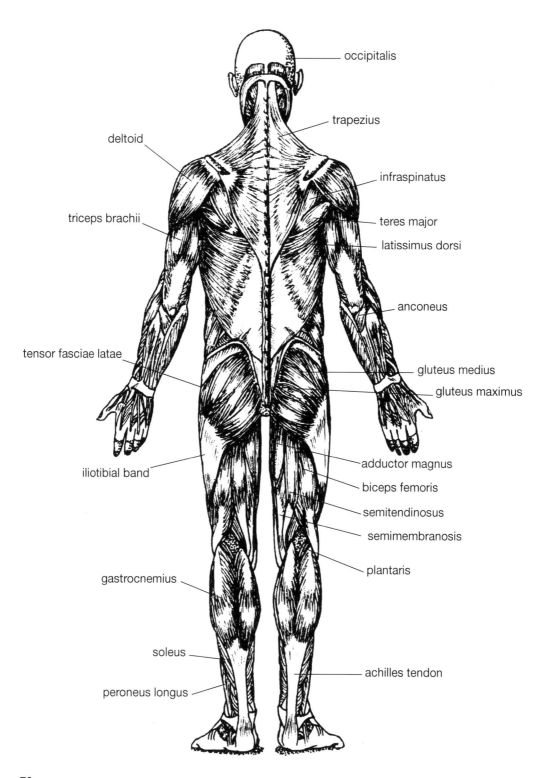

occipitalis

trapezius

deltoid

infraspinatus

triceps brachii

teres major

latissimus dorsi

anconeus

tensor fasciae latae

gluteus medius

gluteus maximus

iliotibial band

adductor magnus

biceps femoris

semitendinosus

semimembranosis

plantaris

gastrocnemius

soleus

achilles tendon

peroneus longus

Achilles Tendon
(Tendo Calcaneus)

Common tendon of the soleus plantaris and gastrocnemius muscles. It is the thickest and strongest tendon of the body.

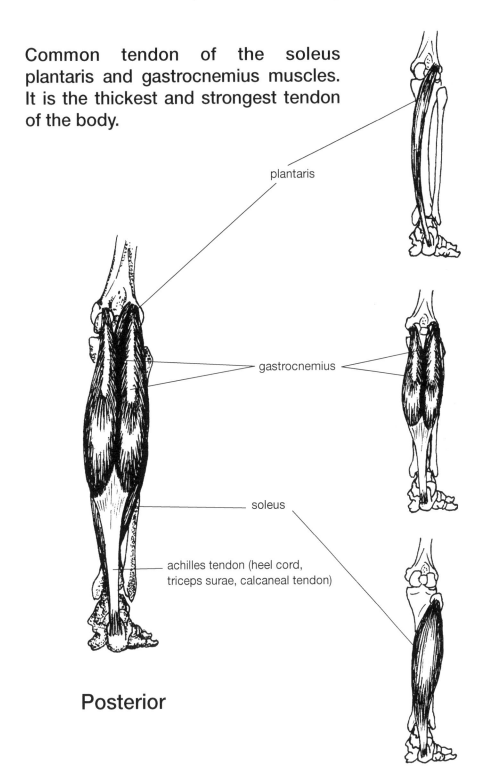

plantaris

gastrocnemius

soleus

achilles tendon (heel cord, triceps surae, calcaneal tendon)

Posterior

Musculotendinous
or
Rotator Cuffs
(Four Short Muscles of the Shoulder)

Anterior

Posterior

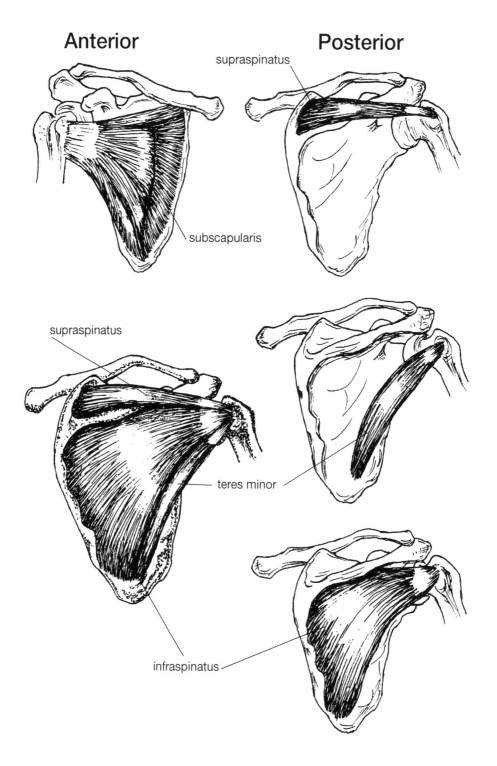

supraspinatus

subscapularis

supraspinatus

teres minor

infraspinatus

Quadriceps Group
of
Thigh (Anterior) Muscles

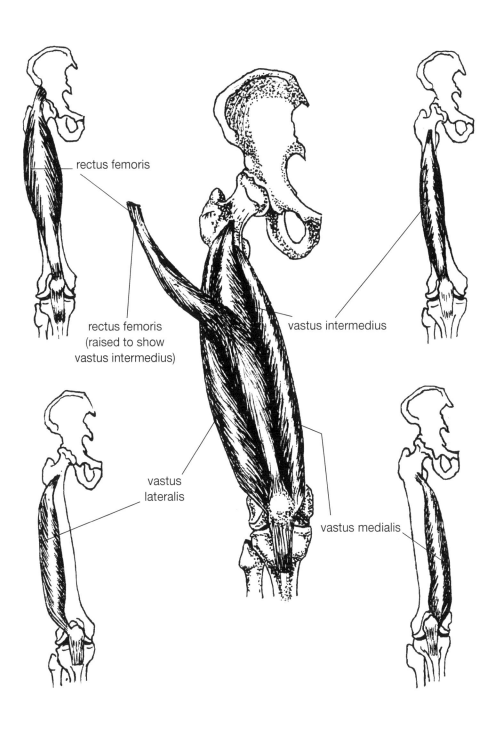

rectus femoris

rectus femoris
(raised to show
vastus intermedius)

vastus intermedius

vastus
lateralis

vastus medialis

Hamstring (Thigh) Muscles

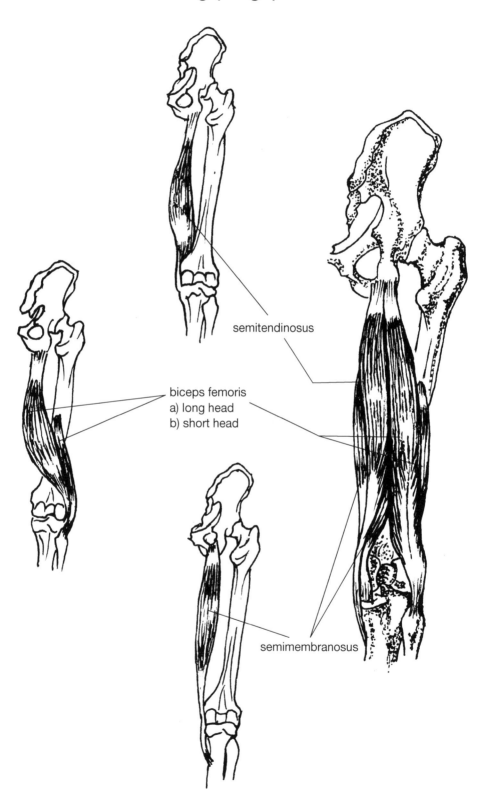

semitendinosus

biceps femoris
a) long head
b) short head

semimembranosus

CHAPTER 4
CASTING

Casts

HISTORY

Plaster of Paris when mixed with water rapidly swells to forms a rigid crystalline structure. During the initial stages of this reaction, the plaster remains in a semi-solid state and may be molded to any desired form. It has been known for centuries that plaster can be manipulated to any shape. Around 1000 AD, the Arabs were the first to use plaster for medicinal purposes to immobilize the affected area.

Plaster casts were first applied by pouring liquid plaster around the limb in an enclosed container. The hardened material conformed to the part and provided immobilization. Later, during the setting process, semi-solid plaster was spread and molded around the part. Many people today believe this to be the method of cast application.

Antonius Mathyson, a Dutch Army surgeon, developed the plaster of Paris bandage in 1852. He dusted powdered plaster into gauze bandages, and the bandages acted as a carrier for the powder plaster. The prepared bandages were then saturated with water and applied to the part in multiple layers. This method facilitated application and resulted in a solid rigid cast. Today, the plaster is no longer merely dusted on the gauze, but rather, various adhesives are utilized to bind the material to the cloth. The use of adhesives prevents the loss of plaster when handling dry bandages and controls the release of the plaster during immersion.

CAST SETTING

The **setting** of a cast is the change of plaster of Paris to crystalline gypsum. The dipping of the bandages releases the plaster from the carrier fabric; this occurs primarily after the application. The layers of plaster react with each other through the gauze, creating a rigid unlaminated piece of gypsum. Any motion during the setting time will create shorter, less rigidly joined, crystals, thus resulting in a weaker cast.

The time interval for plaster of Paris to form a rigid dressing after contact with water is known as the **setting time**. The difference in setting times becomes significant only in terms of personal preference and adeptness of the operator. The cast should be applied rapidly enough to set as one unit. Various factors influence the speed of this reaction. Finely pulverized plaster combines more rapidly with water than do larger granules.

Warm or hot water speeds the chemical reaction. Plaster bandages that are thoroughly squeezed of excess water prior to application are said to set faster. If the dripping water contains residual gypsum from a previous use, the reaction process will be accelerated. Other substances also act as accelerators or retarders when added to the immersion water; however, chemicals usually decrease the strength of the cast.

Commercially available plaster bandages usually fall into two categories: the fast-setting plaster, which hardens in 3 to 5 minutes, and the extra-fast bandages, requiring only 2 to 4 minutes.

GREEN STAGE

A plaster cast that has just settled is in the **green** stage. The chemical reaction in the plaster of Paris is promoted by an abundance of water; however, the water does not completely bind in the crystalline latticework. The excess water accumulates in the pockets, which explains the dampness and the increased weight of the green cast. Maximum cast strength requires evaporation of the unbound water.

CAST DRYING

The cast dries as excess water is evaporated, resulting in a mature cast containing multiple air pockets that lighten the cast and make it permeable. The skin "breathes" through these air vents in the plaster bandage. The drying time for a cast depends on the amount of water to be evaporated and the thickness of the plaster. A thin cast reaches maturity more rapidly than a thicker cast. Evaporation is also promoted or retarded by the surrounding environment. A green cast in a humid atmosphere created by a covering blanket dries slowly. The moisture evaporates more rapidly if the cast is exposed to dry, warm, circulating air. All green casts should be kept uncovered until dry.

CASTING SKILLS

It can be argued that casting can be viewed as an art as well as a medical science. Consequently, it is not the purpose of this book to document the extensive training points of casting methodology, practicing requirements and explanation of the different casting materials.

It should be emphasized that your skills should be developed through learning and practical training under a health care professional, thoroughly experienced in casting procedures and techniques.

As well as plaster casts, there are other types of casts such as synthetic fiberglass and synthetic non-fiberglass. Again, you can learn from an experienced health care professional or you can be trained by a manufacturer's representative.

The most specialized health care professionals devoted to orthopaedic casting are orthopaedic technologists or, depending on the country, orthopaedic technicians. These professionals have usually been formally tested and subsequently certified or registered as qualified orthopaedic technologists or technicians. This qualification confers a wide range of duties and responsibilities, depending on the country – it can mean anything from applying casts to actually being first assistant to the orthopaedic surgeon in the surgical operating room or suite.

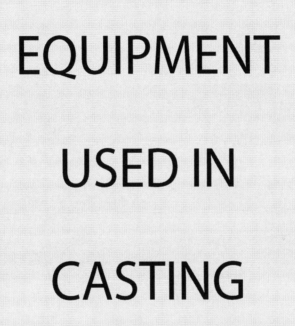

EQUIPMENT

USED IN

CASTING

Methods of Removing Excess Water
From Soaked Plaster Slab

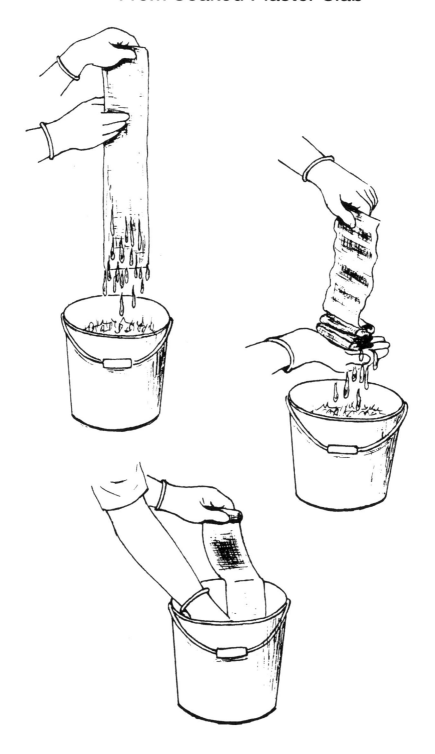

Tools and Equipment

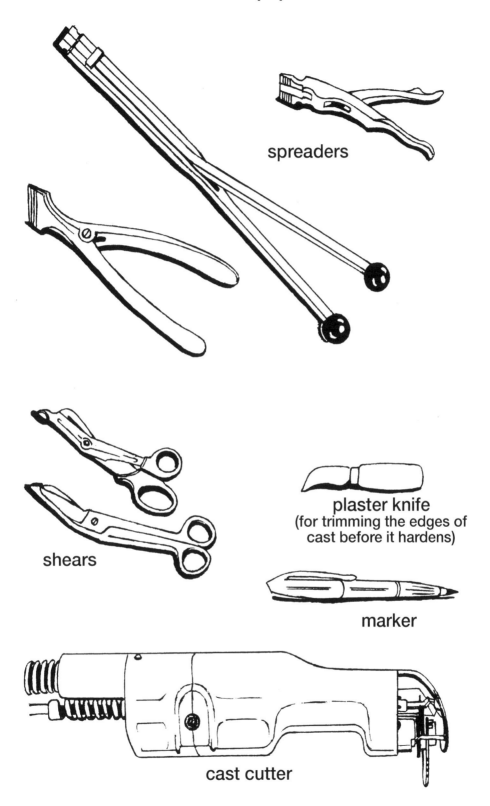

spreaders

shears

plaster knife
(for trimming the edges of
cast before it hardens)

marker

cast cutter

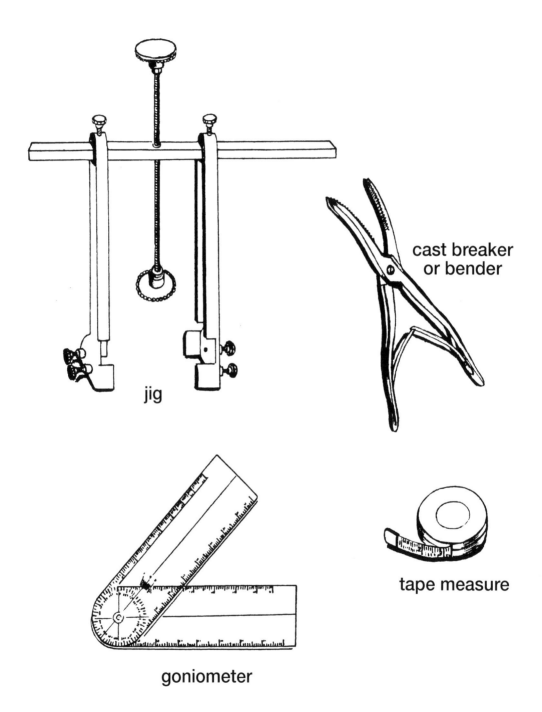

jig

cast breaker
or bender

goniometer

tape measure

Types of Cast Immobilization

Cast immobilization may involve the following anatomic areas: **upper extremities, lower extremities**, **cervical region, spinal (vertebrae)**, or **hip and shoulder areas** (called **spica**), which incorporates the limbs and portions of the trunk.

BODY CAST

A body cast – a circumferential cast enclosing the trunk of the body – may extend from the head or upper chest to the groin or thigh. This type of cast immobilization is used in treating diseases of the cervical, thoracic and lumbar spines such as **fractures** and **scoliosis**, or it may be applied following some types of surgery on the spine. There are several types of body casts.

SPICA CAST

A spica cast is used to immobilize an appendage by incorporating a part of the body proximal to that appendage. The most common spica casts are hip, thumb, and shoulder spicas.

UPPER LIMB CASTS

• **Arm cylinder cast:** Long arm cast with the elbow flexed and the wrist free.

• **Gauntlet cast:** Short cast extending from slightly above or proximal to the wrist to some point in the palm; usually has some outrigger to control one or more digits; used for metacarpal and phalangeal fractures or dislocation.

• **Hanging arm cast:** Long arm cast that, through suspension from a sling around the neck, brings about traction of fracture fragments of the humerus.

• **Short arm cast (SAC):** Below elbow cast mainly used for Colles or wrist fractures; runs from proximal third down to the metacarpophalangeal (MP) joint with the thumb free.

- **Long arm cast (LAC):** Cast extending from the palm and wrist to the axilla, preventing movement at the elbow; used in the treatment of fractures of the forearm, elbow and humerus.

- **Shoulder spica (Airplane cast):** Cast that incorporates the upper torso and envelopes al or a part of the extremity in a position of abduction; used for proximal humeral fractures and rotator cuff tears. Note: sometimes used for a clavicle fractures.

- **Thumb spica:** Below elbow cast that incorporates the thumb; used in treatment of scaphoid (navicular) and the base of the first metacarpal (Bennett's) fractures.

LOWER LIMB CASTS
- **Hip spica:** Cast incorporating the lower torso and extending to one or both lower extremities; used in treatment of femoral fractures, pelvic fractures and for abduction to assist in ambulation for LeggPerthes disease (Petrie spica cast) broomstick.

- **Long leg cast (LAC):** Nonweight bearing cast extending from the upper thigh to the toes; most commonly used for fractures of the tibia and fibula or ligamentous injuries of the knee.

- **Longleg walking cast (LLWC):** Cast from the upper thigh to the toes, with an attached rubber sole device called a walker or cast boot.

- **Quengle cast (Knee brace):** For flexion contracture of the knee, a twopart cast hinged at the knee level, with the lower end of the cast ending at the ankle or foot, and the ankle or foot, and the above knee portion ending at the upper thigh.

- **Cylinder cast (Stove pipe):** Cast from proximal thigh to just above the ankle, most commonly used for injuries of the knee.

- **Short leg cast (SLC):** Nonweight bearing cast extending from just below the knee to the metatarsophalangeal joint; used in injuries of the ankle and foot.

- **Short leg walking cast (SLWC):** Cast with an attached rubber walker or reinforced to accept a cast shoe used for ankle and foot injuries.

- **Patella tendon weightbearing cast (PTB; also known as Sarmiento cast):** Short leg cast with a special feature high condylar wing to reduce rotation and molding about the distal part of the patella; used for management of tibial fractures.

- **Bunion boots:** Cast incorporating the foot just below the malleoli right up to the distal phalanges; used as a rigid postoperative immobilization following bunion surgery.

OTHER CAST TERMS
- **Bivalve cast:** Cast that is split in half by cuts made on opposite sides of the cast to release pressure.

- **Cast boot:** Rubber and canvas device that looks like a large shoe, which can fit over the end of a cast for walking; also called cast shoe or plaster boot.

- **Walker (Walking heel):** Hard rubber wedge directly incorporated into the sole of a cast to allow walking or resting the leg on the ground.

- **Wedge:** Circumferential cutting of the cast and reapplication of plaster over the same cast after a manipulation has been performed to change bony position.

- **Window:** Removal of a piece of cast, usually square or rectangular, to allow inspection of a wound or relieve pressure at a specific point.

NOTES

CHAPTER 5
CAST
COMPLICATIONS

Cast Complications

There are numerous complications due to cast treatment. The related terms are listed here in conjunction with the description of cast treatment and application:

☞ **Burns:** Applying casting material with water temperature too warm, added to the crystallization process that produces heat, can produce skin burns.

☞ **Constrictive edema (also called compartment syndrome):** Disruption of normal venous drainage with resulting fluid accumulation in soft tissue and swelling distal to the point of constriction caused by circulatory embarrassment.

☞ **Decubitus ulcer (also called pressure sore):** An area of pressure necrosis caused by patient lying in same position; also results from continuous or uneven pressure applied with continued immobilization; commonly occurs at the rims of cast and heel.

☞ **Drop foot:** Term applied to paralysis of the peroneal nerve resulting from pressure over the fibular head with inability to dorsiflex the ankle.

☞ **Pin tract infection:** Direct bacterial contamination of area where pins have been used for external traction or skeletal fixation; could potentially lead to osteomyelitis (inflammation of the bone marrow).

☞ **Pressure sore (also called decubitus ulcer):** Breakdown of skin and or subcutaneous tissue because of direct pressure of displaced or bunched cotton padding under cast creating pressure lasting usually in excess of 4 hours; often caused by patient inserting object in cast to reach an area that is itching from plaster dust in cast.

☞ **Superior mesenteric artery syndrome (also called cast syndrome):** Disruption of circulation to the bowel commonly occurring following application of body cast, resulting in abdominal pain, diarrhea; if unrecognized, severe problems occur.

PRESSURE:

☞ **Skin.** A superficial examination of the human body from head to toe reveals many bony prominences which are subcutaneous and are slightly protected by overlying soft tissue. Cast pressure in this area compresses the skin and subcutaneous tissue directly against the underlying bone, causing a localized **ischaemia** (attrition of the tendon). Continued ischaemia results in tissue necrosis and the development of a decubitus ulcer. Originally, the area of compression may cause pain; however, with tissue death, nerves are devitalized and the patient loses his symptoms. If a patient is immobilized in a body or spica cast, certain anatomic locations support most of the body weight. Molding of the plaster may not be sufficient to relieve this local pressure.

☞ **Nerves.** Pressure sores are not the only complications of a poorly padded or improperly molded cast. A superficial peripheral nerve may be compressed by the cast against an underlying bone. The common peroneal nerve may be compressed by plaster at the point where the nerve is subcutaneous, adjacent to bone, and swings around the neck of the fibula. This damage prevents the transmission of nerve impulses and results in anesthesia and paralysis. A complete common peroneal palsy is manifested by a "foot drop" and a loss of sensation on the dorsolateral aspect of the foot. Neurologic damage may be complete or incomplete, and reversible or not. As soon as a neurologic deficit is recognized, the compression on the nerves must be relieved by windowing the cast. Occasionally, the nerve function returns. This may occur because the nerves in the **peripheral nervous system** are surrounded by cellular sheaths which allow them to regenerate. Still, this is not uniformly the case, and permanent palsy may persist. Careful padding and molding of the plaster will prevent this serious complication. The anatomic location of the peroneal nerve must be considered during the application of the lower extremity casts.

CONSTRICTION

☞ Constriction of a limb is caused by a circumferential rigid pressure applied to the extremity from the cast, sufficient to impede or prevent the venous and arterial circulation. When the venous return is diminished and the arterial flow continues, the distal extremity will become swollen and engorged with blood. If the arterial supply is embarrassed or stopped, the distal limb is rendered ischemic and the stage is set for gangrene.

☞ Constriction may result from improper plaster application. A plaster bandage that is cinched or pulled snugly around a limb may constrict the part. The carrier fabric or **mesh** is rigid and creates a binding force when combined with the plaster (gypsum) as it sets. The plaster must be applied without tension. If the position of the limb is altered during cast application, the existing plaster may be sufficiently set to constrict. This is particularly true if the joint angle is changed at an area where two parts of a cast are to be joined, such as the elbow and knee. The limb should not be moved until the entire cast has been applied.

☞ The most common cause of constriction is swelling of the limb after cast application. An injured extremity swells for the first 12 to 24 hours. Treatment, regardless of type, usually increases soft tissue expansion. If a circular cast is applied prior to maximum tissue reaction, continued swelling against the rigid plaster may occlude venous and arterial flow. This possibility exists after circular plaster application for any injury or surgery of the extremities. Constriction may be caused by bloodsoaked and clotted dressings under the plaster binding the limb tightly and thus occluding the circulation. These types of circulatory embarrassment may be prevented if the post injury or postoperative cast is loose enough to permit any swelling that might develop. Unfortunately, excessive looseness of the plaster may defeat the goal of immobilization. An alternative to avoid some of the hazards of constriction is the posterior splint or half cast, which rigidly splints only one side of the extremity. Immobilization is less adequate but the risk of constriction is reduced. One side of the limb may swell without restriction from plaster.

☞ **Recognition of Constriction.** Despite thoughtful and careful technique, constriction does occur, producing distal ischemia. If circulatory embarrassment is recognized early and immediately corrected, no permanent damage may occur. Arterial blood flow to a limb may be completely interrupted for 2 to 4 hours without any residual effects. If the complication resumes, unnoticed, disastrous results may occur.

☞ The recognition of constriction begins with the suspicion. The diagnosis is confirmed by subjective and objective findings. The following six P's are a valuable checklist:

• **Pain:** This is the prime symptom of developing circulatory embarrassment from a cast. The patient's complaints are usually out of proportion to those anticipated after a particular injury or surgery. The pain is burning or cramping in quality and is not localized. A lack of excessive pain should not dismiss constrictive phenomena, for a patient's symptoms may be masked by analgesias or he may demonstrate a high threshold of pain. The evaluation of pain must be individualized.

• **Paraesthesia:** The patient may complain of numbness of the exposed fingers or toes. The sensation may be prickly, tingling, or burning of a quality consistent with paraesthesia.

• **Paralysis:** The patient may or may not be aware of the inability to move his fingers or toes. Severe pain may act to inhibit any attempt at motion. Paralysis may be both a symptom and a sign.

• **Pulseless:** A cardinal finding of interrupted arterial blood flow to the limb is a loss of the peripheral pulses. The **radial** pulse at the wrist and the **dorsalis pedis** pulse on the dorsum of the foot are the usual indicators for the upper and lower extremities. The plaster cast frequently covers these sites and prevents monitoring. If vascular embarrassment is suspected, these areas should be windowed to allow for palpation of the vessels. Circulation is also assessed by the phenomenon of capillary refill in nail beds of the toes or fingers.

Gentle pressure on the nail bed will cause blanching. Upon removal of the pressure, the rapidity with which the nail bed returns to its normal color is an indication of the adequacy of circulation. The normal, uninjured area permits comparison to determine vascular sufficiency. A pulseless limb may demonstrate inadequate capillary refill in the nail beds.

• **Pallor and poikilothermia:** The exposed fingers and toes are pale and cool as a result of arterial insufficiency. This will be evident by examining the opposite side visually and by touch. The digits may have decreased the sensation to pinprick and light touch. **Hypaesthesia** and **anesthesia** are ominous signs.

• **Paralysis:** Motor paralysis is a local finding in the **ischemic** limb. The patient becomes incapable of actively moving his fingers or toes. Paralysis may be due to primary nerve injury; however, in this instance, the other signs of vascular embarrassment are not present. Gentle passive motion of the fingers and toes is exquisitely painful in the ischemic limb. A certain amount of discomfort is anticipated with such a maneuver; however, if the pain is severe, vascular impairment must be considered.

☞ **Correction of Constriction.** A prolonged circulatory insufficiency may result in amputation or the irreversible tissue damage of a **Volkmann's ischemic contracture**, a severe deformity and crippling condition of the hand and arm, also known as **claw hand deformity**. Constriction of a limb by a rigid cast or dressing must be relieved immediately by removing the cast and the division of all padding and dressings down to the skin. A cast may be bivalved and spread; however, if the padding is not divided, it may constrict. Splitting a cast unnecessarily is better than failing to relieve constriction on a limb with circulatory difficulty. A limb has never been lost by splitting the cast and bandage and relieving the pressure. If removal of the cast does not promptly improve circulation, further investigation, and possibly surgery, may become necessary.

In summary, there is first the suspicion, then the observation and the recognition, and finally the prompt action to relieve compression.

CHAPTER 6
TYPES AND CLASSIFICATIONS OF FRACTURES

Classification of Long Bone Injury Location

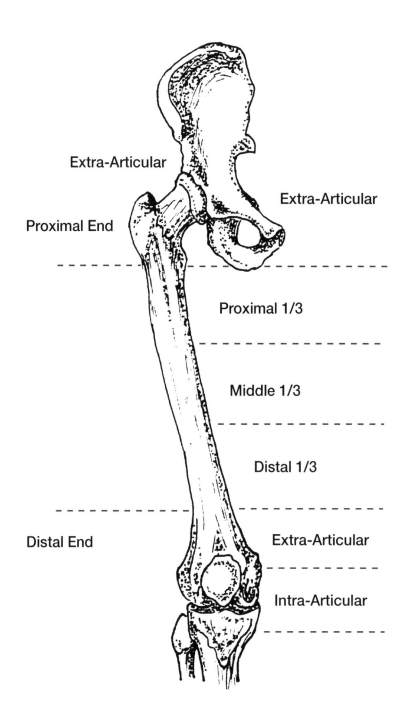

Extra-Articular

Extra-Articular

Proximal End

Proximal 1/3

Middle 1/3

Distal 1/3

Distal End

Extra-Articular

Intra-Articular

Classification of
Fracture Alignment

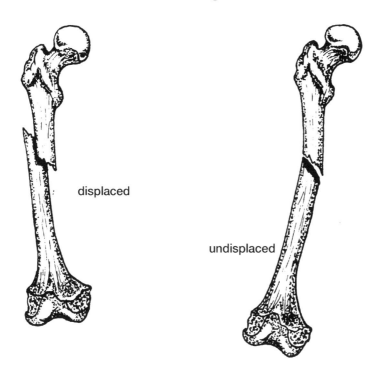

displaced

undisplaced

Classification of
Fracture Type

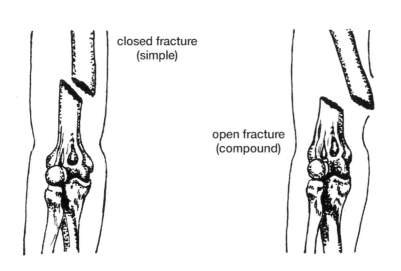

closed fracture
(simple)

open fracture
(compound)

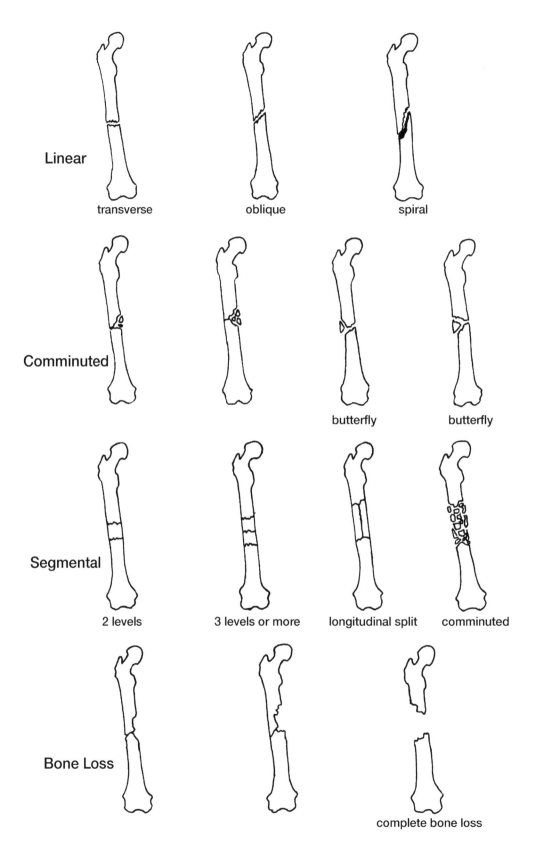

Linear

transverse   oblique   spiral

Comminuted

butterfly   butterfly

Segmental

2 levels   3 levels or more   longitudinal split   comminuted

Bone Loss

complete bone loss

Fracture of the Middle Clavicle
(Sternal End)

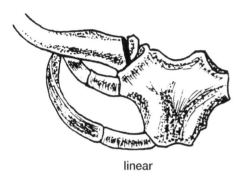

linear

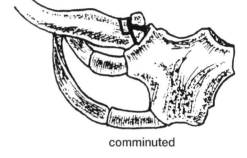

comminuted

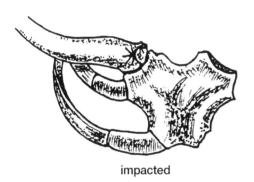

impacted

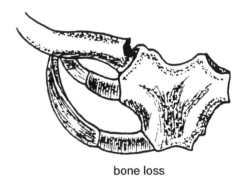

bone loss

Fracture of the Scapula
Extra-Articular (Glenoid Neck)

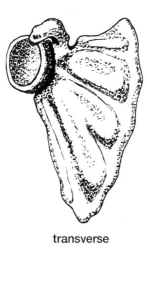

transverse

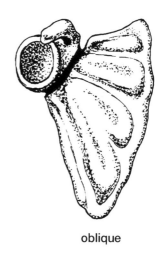

oblique

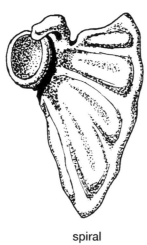

spiral

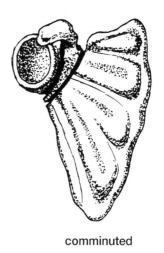

comminuted

Fracture of Scapula
Extra-Articular (Body)

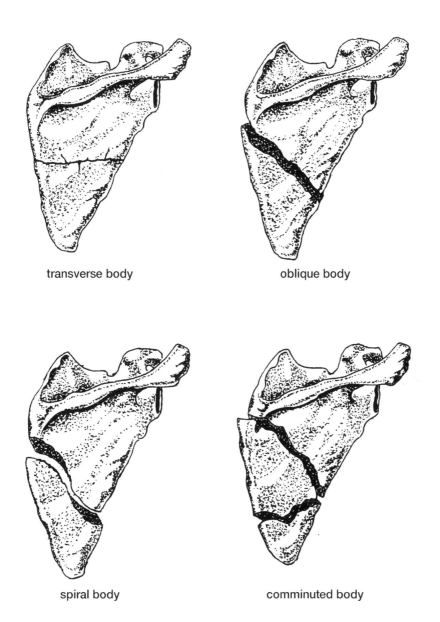

transverse body

oblique body

spiral body

comminuted body

Sternal Joint Injury

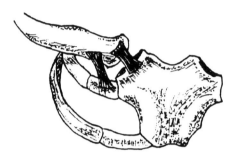

sternoclavicular sprain

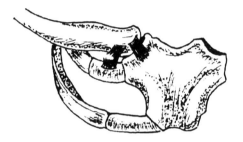

sternoclavicular subluxation

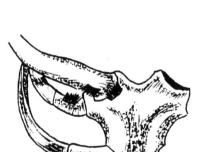

sternoclavicular
dislocation (anterior)

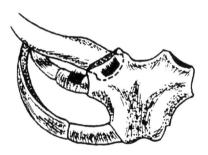

sternoclavicular
dislocation (posterior)

Fracture of the Lateral Clavicle
(Acromial End)

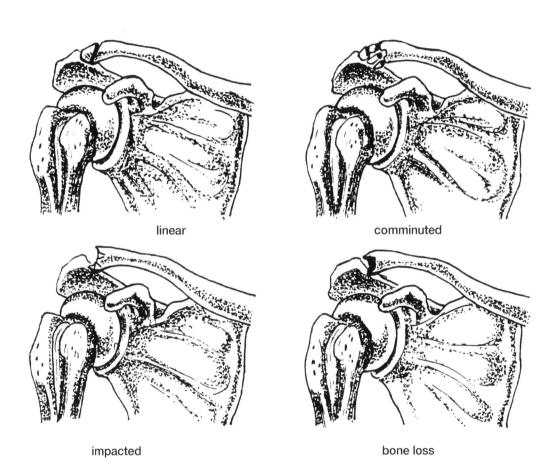

linear

comminuted

impacted

bone loss

Shoulder Joint Injury
(Acromioclavicular)

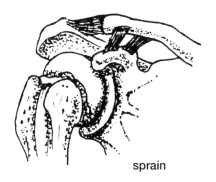

sprain

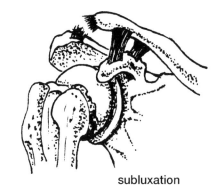

subluxation

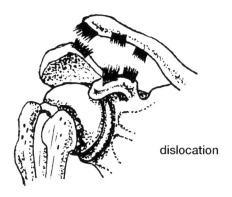

dislocation

Shoulder Joint Injury
(Continued)

Glenohumeral

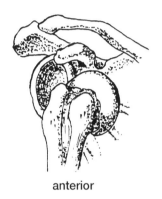

anterior

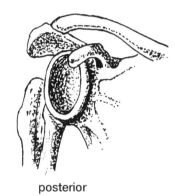

posterior

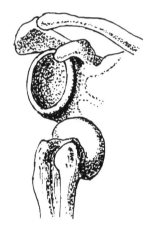

inferior

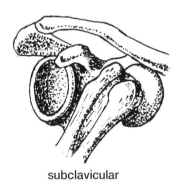

subclavicular

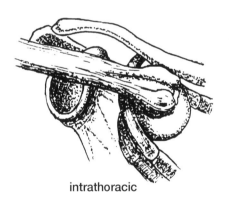

intrathoracic

Fracture of the Proximal Humerus
(Head and Neck)

Intra-Articular (Head)

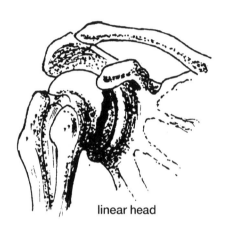

linear head

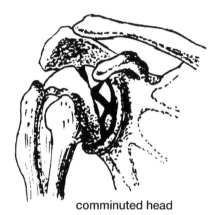

comminuted head

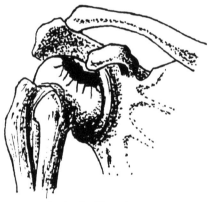

impacted head

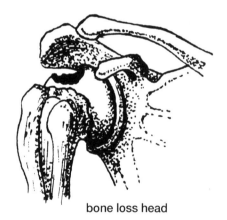

bone loss head

Fracture of the Proximal Humerus
(Head and Neck)

Extra-Articular
(Necks and Tuberosites)

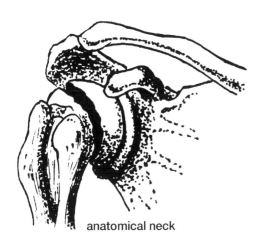

anatomical neck

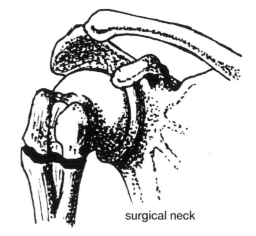

surgical neck

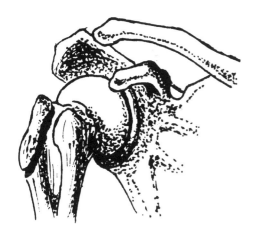

greater tuberosity

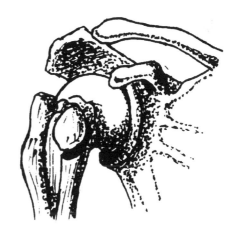

lesser tuberosity

Fracture of the Proximal Humerus

Combinations

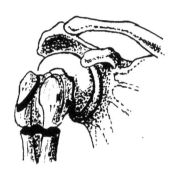 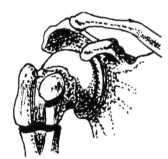 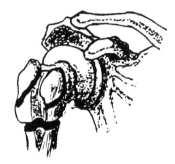

surgical neck with
greater tuberosity

surgical neck with
lesser tuberosity

surgical neck with
greater and lesser
tuberosity

Fracture of the Humeral Shaft

Linear

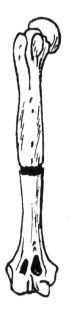 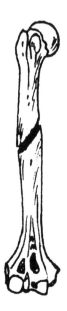 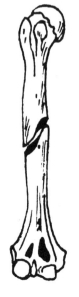

transverse

oblique

spiral

Fracture of the Humeral Shaft
(Continued)

Comminuted

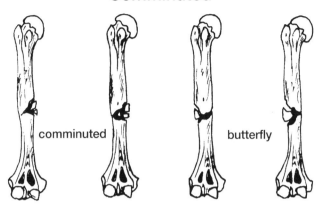

comminuted   butterfly

Segmental

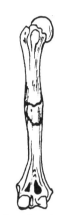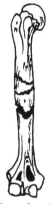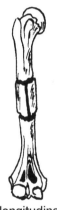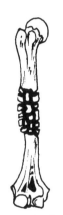

two levels   three levels   longitudinal   comminuted
                or more   split

Bone Loss

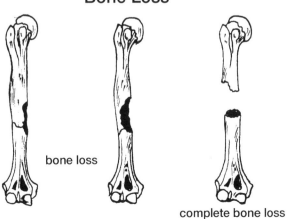

bone loss

complete bone loss

Fracture of the Distal Humerus

Intra-Articular

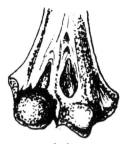

capitulum

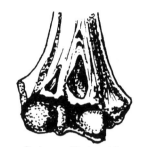

capitulum with trochlea

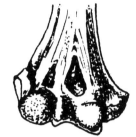

lateral epicondyle

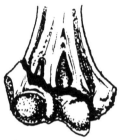

lateral epicondyle
with trochlea

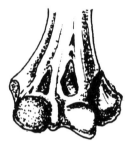

medial epicondyle

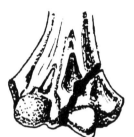

medial epicondyle
with trochlea

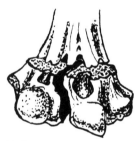

T-shaped intercondylar with
separation of the fragments
and significant rotary
deformity

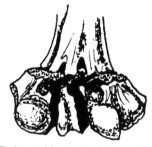

T-shaped intercondylar with
severe comminution of the
articular surface

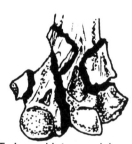

T-shaped intercondylar
with severe comminution of
the shaft

Extra-Articular

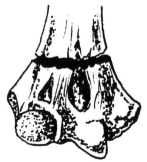

supracondylar

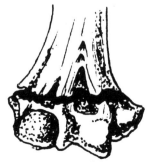

transcondylar

Elbow Joint Injury

Radio-Ulnar-Humeral Dislocation

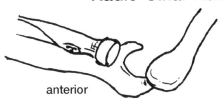

anterior

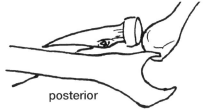

posterior

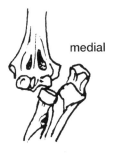

medial

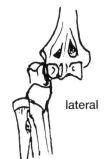

lateral

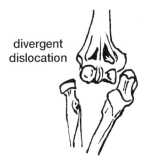

divergent dislocation

Radial Head
(Proximal Radio-Ulnar/Radio-Humeral)
Dislocation

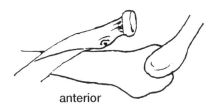

anterior

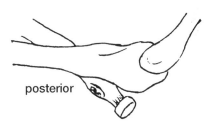

posterior

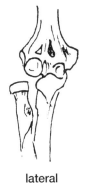

lateral

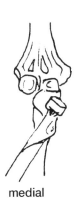

medial

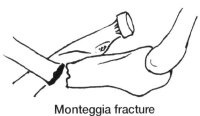

Monteggia fracture

Fracture of the Proximal Ulna
(Coronoid/Olecranon)

Intra-Articular
(Trochlear Notch)

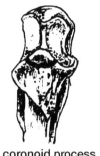

coronoid process

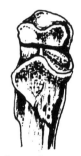

linear fracture

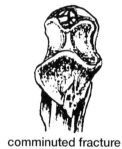

comminuted fracture
olecranon process

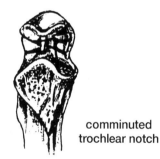

comminuted
trochlear notch

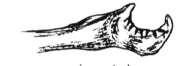

impacted

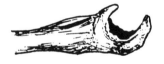

articular bone loss

Fracture of the Patella

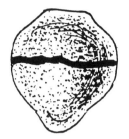

linear
(transverse)

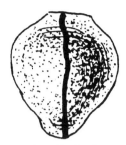

longitudinal

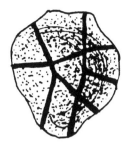

comminuted

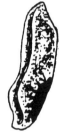

impacted

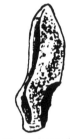

articular bone loss

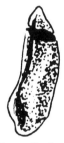

extra-articular

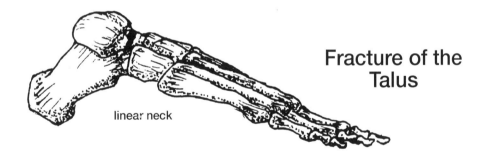

Fracture of the Talus

linear neck

Fracture of the Calcaneus
(Os Calcis)

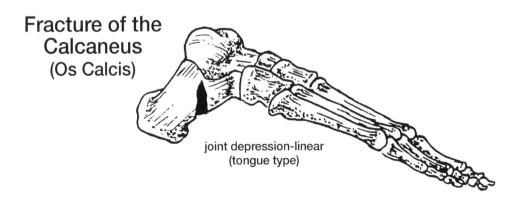

joint depression-linear
(tongue type)

Foot Joint Injury

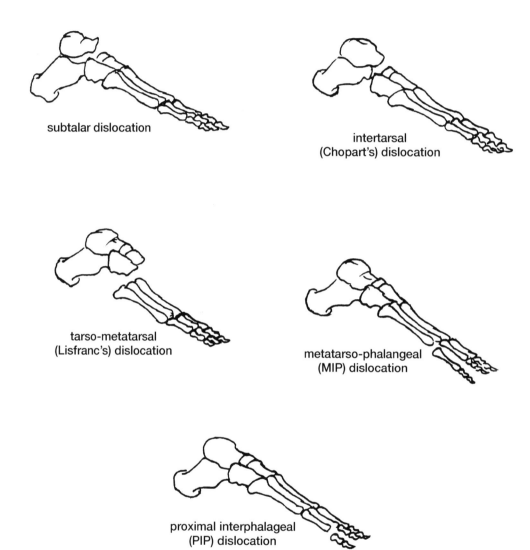

subtalar dislocation

intertarsal
(Chopart's) dislocation

tarso-metatarsal
(Lisfranc's) dislocation

metatarso-phalangeal
(MIP) dislocation

proximal interphalageal
(PIP) dislocation

Knee Joint Injury

Patello-Femoral (Patella) Dislocation

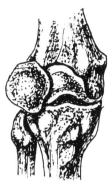

lateral
subluxation

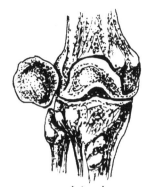

lateral
dislocation

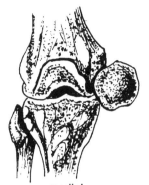

medial
dislocation

Tibio-Femoral Dislocation

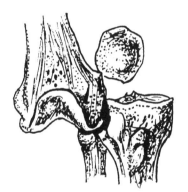

posterior

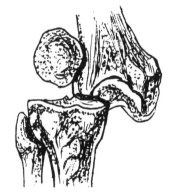

anterior

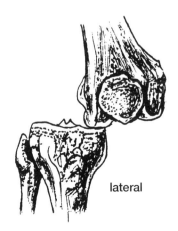

lateral

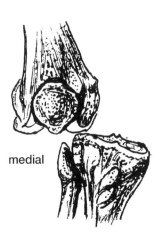

medial

Fracture of the Proximal Tibia
(Tibial Plateau)

Isolated Intra-Articular

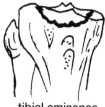

tibial eminence

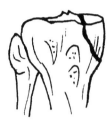

linear plateau

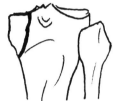

linear posterior

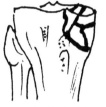

comminuted plateau

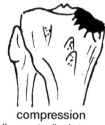

compression
(impacted) plateau

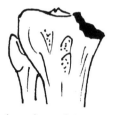

boneless plateau

Combination Intra-Articular

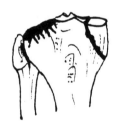

linear and
compression (impacted)
separate plateaus

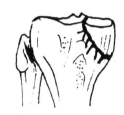

linear compression
(impacted) isolated plateau

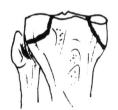

bi-condylar linear
both plateaus

Extra-Articular

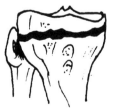

linear metaphysis

Ankle Fractures

Internal Rotation/Adduction

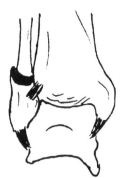

Weber A-transverse
fracture fibula distal to
tibio-fibular ligament

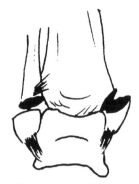

Weber A-bimalleolar
fracture transverse
laterally, oblique medially

External Rotation/Abduction

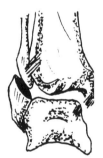

Weber B-oblique fracture
fibula at level of tibio-
fibular ligament, ruptured
deltoid ligament

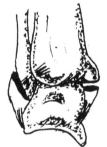

Weber B-bimalleolar
fracture, oblique laterally,
transverse medially

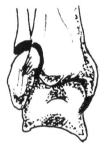

Weber B-fibula fracture
and avulsion of tibio-
fibular ligament

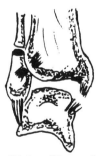

Weber C1-proximal
fibula fracture to
tibio-fibular ligament
and deltoid ligament

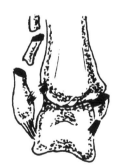

Weber C2-proximal to
tibio-fibular ligament with
syndesmotic disruption

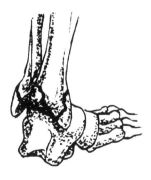

trimalleolar

Fracture of the Mid-Tarsal Bones

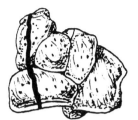

navicular
linear 1st cuneiform

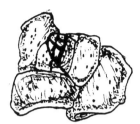

comminuted
2nd cuneiform

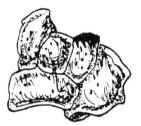

impacted
3rd cuneiform

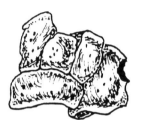

articular bone loss
cuboid

Fracture of the Metatarsal Shaft

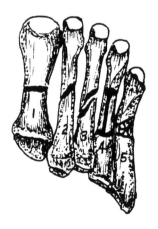

1   transverse
2   oblique
3   spiral
4   longitudinal split
5   comminuted

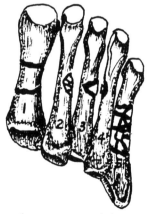

1   segmental
2   comminuted
3   butterfly
4   butterfly
5   comminuted
     segmental

Fracture of the Proximal Radius
(Head and Neck)

Intra-Articular (Head)

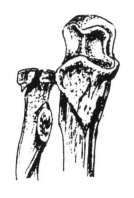

linear

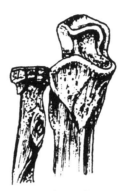

comminuted

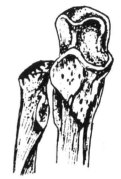

impacted

Extra-Articular (Neck)

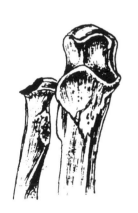

bone loss

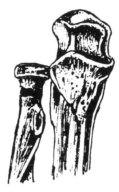

radial neck

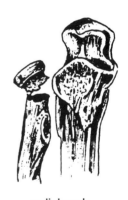

radial neck
with angulation

Fracture of the Distal Radius

Intra-Articular

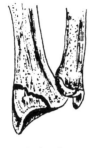

anterior linear

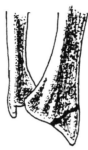

posterior linear

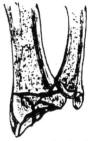

comminuted

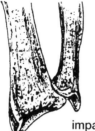

impacted

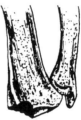

bone loss

Extra-Articular

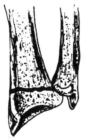

transverse

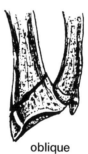

oblique

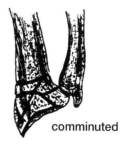

spiral   comminuted

Wrist Joint Injury

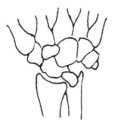

dorsal perilunate
dislocation

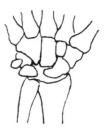

volar lunate
dislocation

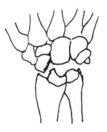

dorsal transscaphoid
perilunate dislocation

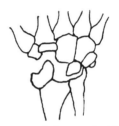

complete scaphoid
perilunate dislocation

Ligament Injuries

normal scapholate
angle 30° - 60°

dorsiflexed intercalated segment
instability (DISI) (dorsal tilt of
lunate) scapholate angle greater
than 70°

volar flexed instrument segment
instability (VISI)(volar tilt of lunate)
scapholate angle 35°

isolated rotarysubluxation of
scaphoid (vertical scaphoid)

119

Fracture of the Carpal Bones

Trapezium

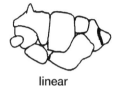 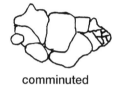 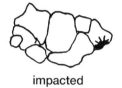 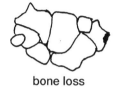

| linear | comminuted | impacted | bone loss |

Scaphoid

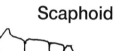 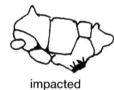 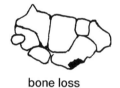

| linear | comminuted | impacted | bone loss |

Trapezoid

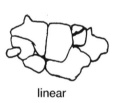 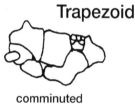 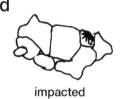 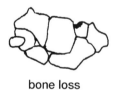

| linear | comminuted | impacted | bone loss |

Capitate

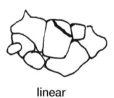 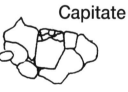 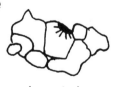 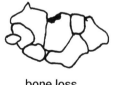

| linear | comminuted | impacted | bone loss |

Fracture of the Carpal Bones
(Continued)

Hamate

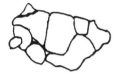
linear

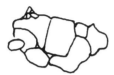
comminuted

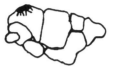
impacted

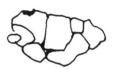
bone loss

Pisiform

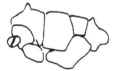
linear

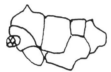
comminuted

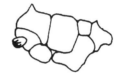
impacted

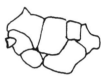
bone loss

Triangular

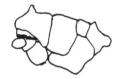
linear

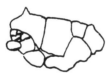
comminuted

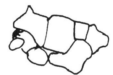
impacted

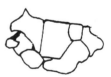
bone loss

Lunate

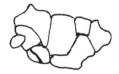
linear

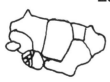
comminuted

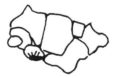
impacted

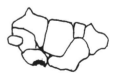
bone loss

Fracture of the Proximal Femur

Extra-Articular

  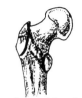

apophyseal fracture
greater trochanter

apophyseal fracture
lesser trochanter

apophyseal fracture
both trochanters

Femoral Neck

Garden 1
incomplete subcapital
fracture without
displacement

 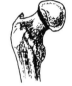

Garden 2
complete subcapital
fracture without
displacement

Garden 3
complete subcapital
fracture with partial
displacement

Garden 4
complete subcapital
fracture with full
displacement

mid-cervical

base of the neck
(pertrochanteric)

Intertrochanteric

two-part fracture along
the intertrochanteric line
without extension below
the lesser trochanter

three-part fracture
including the lesser
trochanter with varus
deformity

three-to-four part
intertrochanteric with
large posterior-medial
comminution

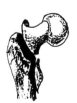 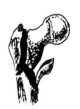

comminuted
intertrochanteric with
oblique subtrochanteric
extension

Fracture of the Distal Femur

Intra-Articular

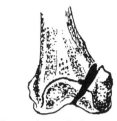

linear through the notch

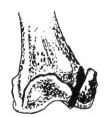

linear through the weight-bearing cartilage

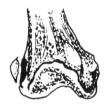

avulsion

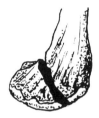

posterior femoral condyle (lateral view)

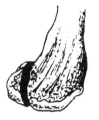

posterior femoral condyle (lateral view)

Extra-Articular

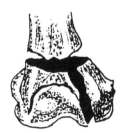

T-shaped through the notch

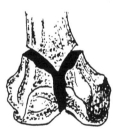

T-shaped through the weight bearing cartilage

Y-shaped through the notch

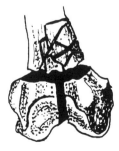

T-shaped with shaft comminution

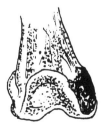

impacted

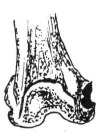

bone loss

Isolated Pelvic Fractures

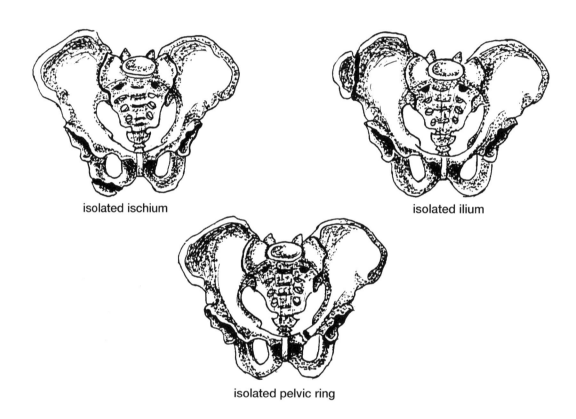

isolated ischium

isolated ilium

isolated pelvic ring

Fracture of the Pelvic Girdle

lateral compression fractures - anterior and posterior fractures or
ligamentous disruption with displacement of one side of the ring
relative to the other side of the sacrum

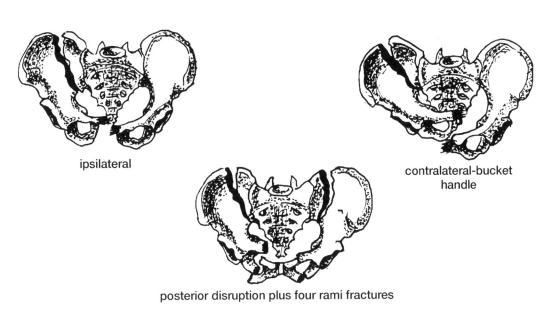

ipsilateral

contralateral-bucket
handle

posterior disruption plus four rami fractures

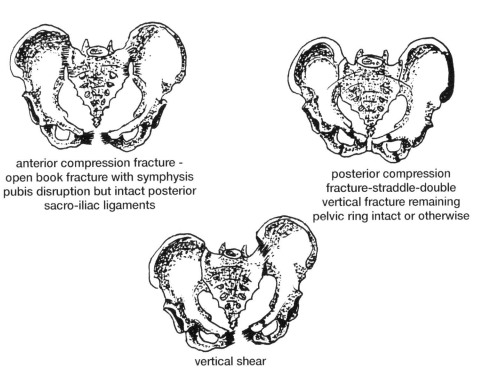

anterior compression fracture -
open book fracture with symphysis
pubis disruption but intact posterior
sacro-iliac ligaments

posterior compression
fracture-straddle-double
vertical fracture remaining
pelvic ring intact or otherwise

vertical shear

Fracture of the Acetabulum

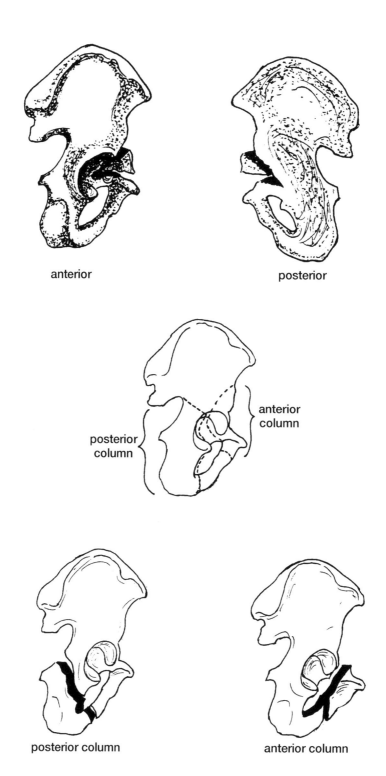

anterior   posterior

posterior
column   anterior
                                      column

posterior column   anterior column

Hip Joint Injury

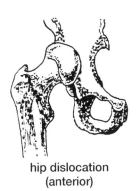

hip dislocation
(anterior)

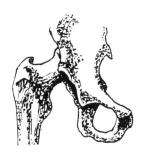

hip dislocation
(posterior)

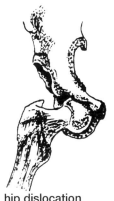

hip dislocation
(obturator)

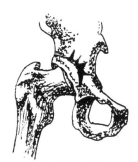

hip dislocation
(central)

Hip Fracture Dislocation
(Epstein)

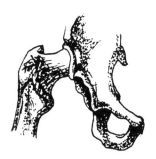

Epstein type 1-
simple dislocation

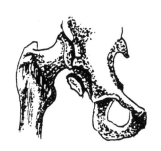

Epstein type 2 - dislocation
with fracture of the
acetabulum

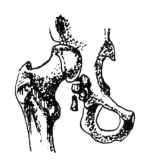

Epstein type 3
- dislocation with
comminuted fracture of
the posterior wall

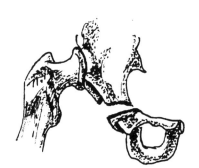

Epstein type 4 - dislocation
with fracture of the
acetabulum

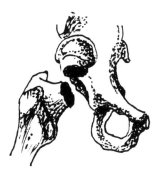

dislocation with fracture of
the femoral neck

Hip Fracture Dislocation
(Pipkin)

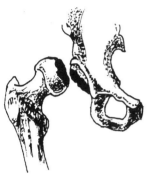

Pipkin type 1 - posterior
dislocation with fracture
of the femoral head
caudal to fovea centralis

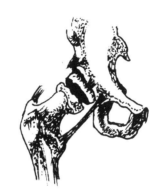

Pipkin type 2 - posterior
with fracture of the
femoral head cephalad
to fovea centralis

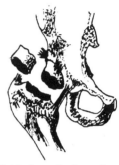

Pipkin type 3 - type 1
or 2 with associated
fracture of the femoral
neck

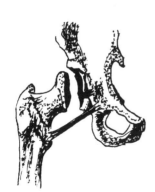

Pipkin type 4 - type 1,
2, or 3 with associated
fracture of the
acetabulum

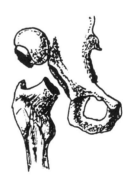

dislocation with fracture
of the neck

Epiphyseal Fractures
(Salter-Harris Classification)

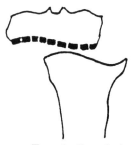

Type 1 - the whole epiphysis is separated from the shaft

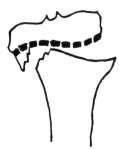

Type 2 - the epiphysis is displaced carrying with it a small triangular metaphyseal fragment (the commonest injury)

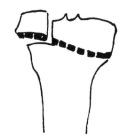

Type 3 - separation of part of the epiphysis

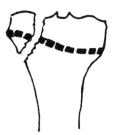

Type 4 - separation of part of the epiphysis with a metaphyseal fragment

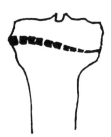

Type 5 - crushing of part of or all of the epiphysis

Thoracic and Lumbar
Spine Injuries

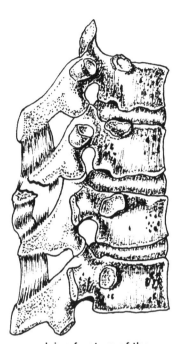

avulsion fracture of the
tip of a spinous process

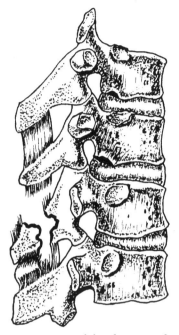

avulsion fracture of a
spinous process

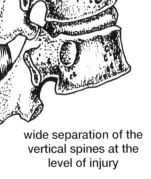

wide separation of the
vertical spines at the
level of injury

NOTES

CHAPTER 7
UPPER EXTREMITY FRACTURES

Colles Fracture

Fractures of the lower end of the **radius** are by far the most common cases which the health care professional will encounter. The majority of all cases are produced by indirect trauma (i.e., a FOOSH – a fall on an outstretched hand). They are seen mainly in middle-aged and elderly women, osteoporosis being the contributory factor.

Abraham Colles of Dublin first described this fracture in 1814. He placed the break 11/2 inches above the carpal articulation; although we now know that the great majority of injuries lie much nearer to the wrist joint than he had conjectured, we continue to refer to the fractures of the lower extremity of the radius by his name.

Diagnosis. Radiographs must be taken in all cases where there is pain in the wrist and tenderness over the distal end of the radius as a result of a fall. The site of maximum tenderness will help to differentiate the fracture of the scaphoid. Where there is marked displacement, the clinical appearance is so characteristic that diagnosis presents no difficulty. In the majority of cases, the fracture is easily identified. Although other injuries in the arm occurring in association with Colles fracture are uncommon, the scaphoid, the elbow and the shoulder should nevertheless be clinically examined and the scaphoid should be carefully scrutinized on the radiograph.

Treatment. Does the fracture require manipulation? If the fracture is grossly displaced, the displacement should be reduced. If undisplaced, no manipulation is needed and conservative treatment entails applying a back slab for 2 to 5 days. This will allow room for any kind of soft tissue swelling. Ask the patient to come back for a new circular cast.

However, if there is greater trauma, and there is a dorsal tilt of the distal fragment, closed manipulation is required. A displacement of the ulnar styloid indicates a serious disruption of the inferior radioulnar

Colle's Fracture

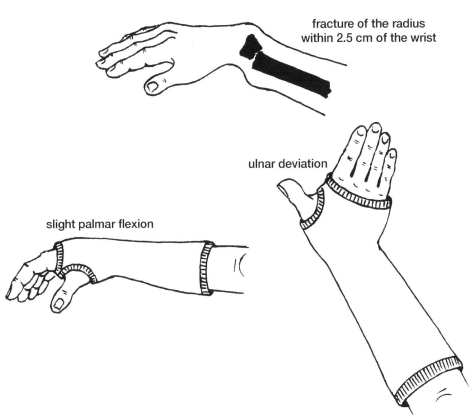

fracture of the radius within 2.5 cm of the wrist

ulnar deviation

slight palmar flexion

Smith's Fracture
(Reverse Colle's Fracture)

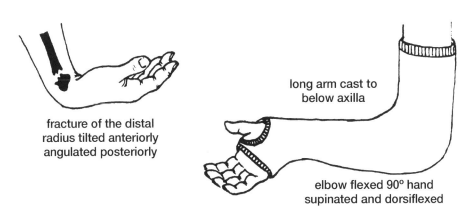

fracture of the distal radius tilted anteriorly angulated posteriorly

long arm cast to below axilla

elbow flexed 90° hand supinated and dorsiflexed

joint. An attempt at correction should be made irrespective of other appearances. Reduction techniques start with the preparation of an ideal plaster back slab. The length should equal the distance of the olecranon to the metacarpal heads.

The first, essential stage in the reduction of Colles fracture is to disimpact the radial fragment. If the post reduction x-ray is acceptable, a sling should be applied above the heart to help reduce swelling. Take care to ensure that there is no constriction of the injured limb. The patient is then shown various finger exercises and is advised of normal plaster care. The patient is seen the next day, and the patient's fingers are examined to assess circulation and the degree of swelling. Thereafter, the patient should be examined within the next 5 days with a view to completion of the plaster.

In some cases, due to inexperience, positional errors occur. The most common fault is the lack of ulnar deviation. Above average displacement will contribute to bone shortening, and the patient will suffer radial deviation. This pattern is sometimes referred to as **Madelung's deformity**, a term initially used to describe a condition occurring in adolescents. Too much wrist flexion could impede the median nerve which would lead to carpal tunnel syndrome.

Two other important complications may arise after the Colles fracture: a delayed rupture of the extensor pollicis longus tendon may occur some months after the injury, the result of ischaemia; and **Sudeck's atrophy** – usually diagnosed some weeks after the cast fixation has been discontinued – which is characterized by marked swelling of the wrist hand and fingers, gross stiffness of the fingers, and carpal decalcification, which is clearly visible on radiographs of the region.

Fracture of the Scaphoid (Navicular)

The scaphoid is the most commonly fractured carpal bone. The injury usually occurs in workingmen, and is generally a result of a blow to the palm of the hand.

Diagnosis. The diagnosis for scaphoid fracture is partly clinical and partly radiological. The main signs are swelling and tenderness in the anatomical snuff box with pain in wrist movements. Radiologically, extra oblique or "scaphoid views" of the wrist are necessary because the fracture may be hairline. If the clinical diagnosis is made and the x-ray is negative, the wrist is immobilized for two weeks; then the area is x-rayed again, when the fracture, if present, will be revealed. Approximately 14 to 17 days is required for the bone to calcify.

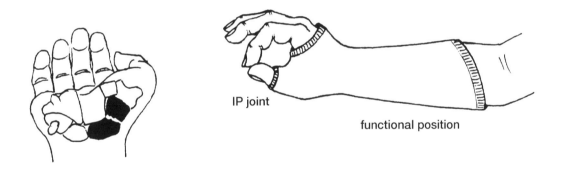

IP joint

functional position

Complications. Fracture through the wrist may deprive the proximal half of the bone of its blood supply, which enters through the distal half. When this occurs, union becomes uncertain and **avascular necrosis** of the proximal fragments may occur causing a degeneration of the wrist. There are three anatomical reasons why fracture of the scaphoid proximal half is susceptible to avascular necrosis: a poor blood supply from the distal to the proximal; an excessive amount of synovial fluid interfering with bone formation, and a poor anatomical position which results in a difficulty to mould.

Treatment. The wrist is immobilized in a scaphoid plaster in a functional position about 10° to 15° dorsiflexion. This will prevent the patient from losing motion of the wrist after the cast is removed. The plaster extends from the proximal third of the forearm to the knuckles including the thumb (interphalangeal joint). This must be continued until the clinical signs disappear, and there is radiological evidence of a union. (At least 6 weeks is required and in some cases, it takes several months.)

A nonunion of the scaphoid fracture may be treated with a bone graft or with a screw placed across the fracture line. Internal fixation is occasionally useful for the severely displaced fresh fracture or a fracture that is associated with a dislocation of the wrist. (An established nonunion or painful ischaemic necrosis may also necessitate surgery. An excision of the necrotic fragment of the radial styloid is more commonly performed than arthrodesis of the wrist).

To prevent **osteoarthritis**, an excision might be considered because a bone that develops avascular necrosis will have an irregular shape, thus creating an attrition towards the surrounding soft tissue. It is worth mentioning, however, that many non-unions remain completely symptom free; discovery may be quite accidental, only occurring when x-raying the wrist for other reasons.

Bennet's Fracture

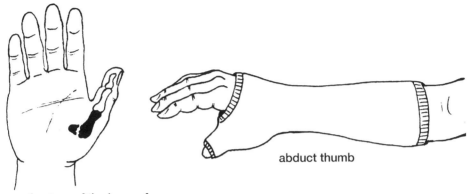

fracture of the base of
the thumb metacarpal

abduct thumb

This is a fracture dislocation of the carpometacarpal joint of the thumb. It can usually be treated by extending the thumb in abduction, applying a plaster cast and exerting pressure on the base of the thumb while the plaster sets. Four to six weeks in plaster is usually sufficient for union. In rare cases, open reduction may be necessary, in which case the fragment is pinned in position. Note the difference between **Rolando's fracture** and Bennet's fracture: Rolando's fracture is a T-shaped intra-articular fracture at the base of the first metacarpal.

Boxer's Fracture

These are common and frequently stable unless grossly displaced. They usually need little manipulation, and immobilization in a plaster cast for 3 to 4 weeks, allowing the hand to be used while union is progressing. A fracture of the neck of the fifth metacarpal (Boxer's) often follows a blow with a clenched fist. The head of the fifth metacarpal is displaced into the palm (anterior tilt), and the patient presents with a flattening or loss of knuckle prominence. An attempt is usually made to reduce it by manipulation. A simple dorsal slab (ulna gutter splint), completed after a few days, may be quite satisfactory. Better fixation is achieved by the addition of a finger extension to the basic slab. Three weeks in a plaster is sufficient.

Note: if there is gross angulation, the MP joint is flexed; pressure is then applied to the head via the proximal phalanx, using the thumb. The fingers apply counter-pressure to the shaft. Reduction is generally easy, but must be maintained during setting of the plaster.

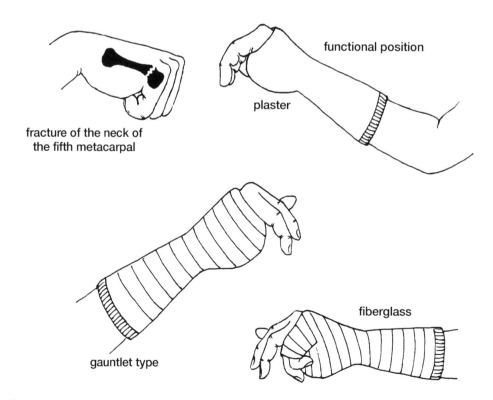

fracture of the neck of
the fifth metacarpal

functional position

plaster

gauntlet type

fiberglass

Fracture of the Shaft of the Humerus

Injury to the humerus may result in a transverse or spiral fracture to the mid-shaft of the bone.

Treatment. Whenever possible, closed reduction is the treatment of choice, using a sugar-tong splint with a collar and cuff, a hanging cast or the less used shoulder spica as the immobilizing agent. If open reduction is deemed necessary, either intramedullary fixation or compression plate fixation is usually employed.

Complications. The two major complications of fractures of the shaft of the humerus are non-union of the bone and radial nerve palsy. Injury to radial nerves adjacent to the musculospiral groove may accompany humeral shaft fractures and may result in the patient losing the power to actively dorsiflex the wrist and extend fingers and thumb metacarpal. The wrist hangs limply in flexed position. The condition is called **wrist drop**. If the radial nerve is only bruised and not severed in association with the humeral shaft fracture, nerve function returns in the majority of patients within 3 to 9 months. The wrist should be splinted in dorsiflexed position (the position of function) while awaiting nerve regeneration.

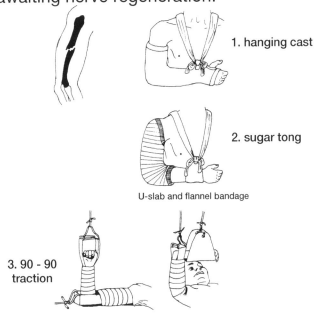

1. hanging cast

2. sugar tong

U-slab and flannel bandage

3. 90 - 90 traction

Supracondylar Fracture of the Humerus

The supracondylar area of the humerus is the lower flared end of the bone just above the elbow joint. According to Gartland, (Fundamentals of Orthopaedics, 1987) fractures through this area occur commonly in children but rarely in adults. A supracondylar fracture is characteristically produced by a fall on the outstretched arm with the elbow in hyperextension; if the fracture is incomplete, there is little deformity. Less than 1% of supracondylar fractures are the reverse, or flexion type, produced by a fall on the flexed elbow with the resulting anterior displacement of the distal fragment. It is an error to confuse the types and to treat in extension the posteriorly displaced distal fragment, with angulation, apex anteriorly. This mistake can cause prolonged hyperextension and limited flexion.

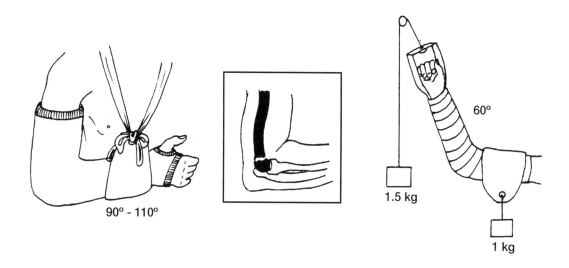

90° - 110°   60°   1.5 kg   1 kg

Treatment. When a supracondylar fracture is seen promptly, before swelling has appeared – even though the displacement is extreme – an excellent result can be obtained by immediate closed reduction and immobilization in flexion. After reduction, the fracture must be maintained in a stable position. Flexion of the elbow stretches the triceps over the fracture, often splinting it most efficiently (posterior displacement). The aim should be to flex the elbow as far as the state of the circulation will permit. Assuming that an 80° pulse is present (if present before the manipulation it should still be there, and if absent it will hopefully have been restored) continue flexion of the elbow until the pulse disappears (due to the elbow flexure crease along with the swelling compressing the brachial artery). In such cases, apply a back slab and sling – never apply a complete plaster because of the risks of swelling.

Complications. Inadequate or incomplete reduction of fracture damage can occur due to nerves passing over the fracture site. Circulatory impairment is heralded by a weak or absent radial pulse. In extreme cases, this can lead to Volkmann's ischemic contracture **(see Chapter 4)**.

Fracture of the Clavical

This is one of the most common fractures occurring in children and young adults. Most clavicular injuries result from a fall on the outstretched hand. In a child, the fracture is usually of the **greenstick** type. The most common fracture sites occur in the middle and outer third junction and throughout the middle third. Subluxations and dislocations, however, may involve the **acromioclavicular** joint and the **sternoclavicular** joint.

Treatment. Treatment for most clavicular fractures (greenstick or undisplaced fractures) consists of supporting the weight of the arm in a broad sling. With the more severely displaced fractures, an attempt is usually made to secure a partial reduction by means of a figure-of-eight bandage but this is not an effective device and may be uncomfortable. Occasionally, internal fixation is required if the displacement is sufficiently severe. The majority of clavicular fractures heal well, give excellent function and after remodeling are cosmetically satisfactory. Three weeks of support is normally sufficient and complications are rare.

Note: The clavicle bone is the last bone to fuse in the skeletal system.

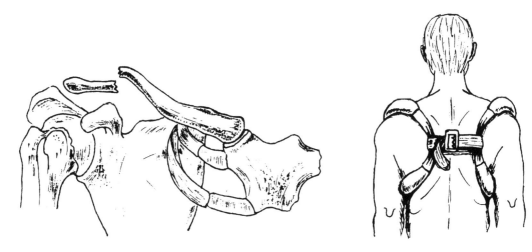

CHAPTER 8
LOWER EXTREMITY FRACTURES

Dislocation of the Hip

In children, traumatic dislocation of the hip is generally the result of a difficult delivery, an athletic injury or a vehicular accident. To dislocate the hip a child requires less force than an adult. Boys are the majority of the patients. The hip is commonly dislocated posteriorly so the leg assumes a characteristic positional deformity of shortening and internal rotation.

There are five types of hip dislocation: **anterior, posterior, superior, inferior** and **central**. The less common anterior dislocation of the femoral head carries with it the threat of impingement against the femoral artery. Note: during hip dislocation, the head of the femur is susceptible to **avascular necrosis** or the later **degenerative arthritis** of the hip. The reason for this is that the **obturator artery,**

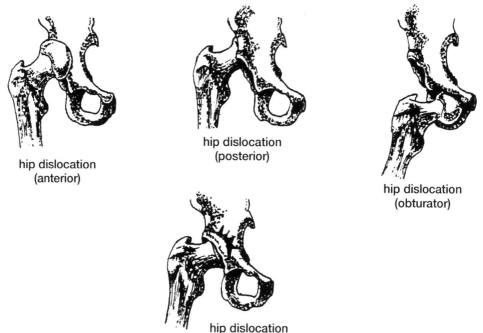

hip dislocation
(anterior)

hip dislocation
(posterior)

hip dislocation
(obturator)

hip dislocation

which supplies a small portion of blood to the head of the femur, will likely be ruptured together with the **ligamentum teres**.

Treatment. Closed manipulative reduction of the dislocation should be carried out promptly, certainly within the first 24 hours following injury. The patient is maintained at bed rest with the injured

146

limb in **Buck's traction** for a period of two weeks. Hip flexion and hip adduction motions should be avoided for a six to eight week period.

The prognosis is good if the injury is not complicated by an associated fracture and treatment has been carried out promptly. The prognosis for future hip function is not good, however, if the dislocation is associated with fracture about the femoral head or **acetabulum**, since this implies more severe trauma to the joint at the time of injury. Open reduction of the fragments may be required.

Hip Fracture Dislocation
(Epstein)

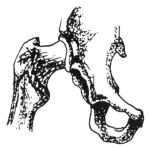

Epstein type 1 -
simple dislocation

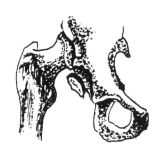

Epstein type 2 -
dislocation with fracture
of the acetabulum

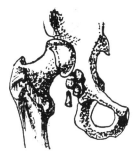

Epstein type 3 -
dislocation with
comminuted fracture of
the posterior wall

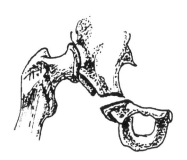

Epstein type 4 -
dislocation with fracture
of the acetabulum

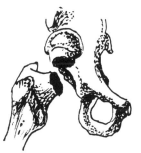

dislocation with fracture of
the femoral neck

Fracture Neck of the Femur

This is a common injury in elderly people, and the bone is frequently **osteoporic**. They are therefore **pathological** fractures. There are four levels (sites) of fractures that are well recognized around the femoral neck: **cersubcapital, transcervical, intertrochanteric (or basal)** and **pretrochanteric** fractures. Diagnosis for this kind of trauma will be the patient's inability to bear weight after a fall, particularly if he or she is elderly. Tenderness will be found over the femoral neck anteriorly. Pain is produced by rotation of the hip. Bruising is a late sign in extra capsular fractures, and is absent in acute injuries and in intracapsular fractures.

Complications. Intracapsular fractures are prone to complications for two clear reasons:

1. The blood supply to the head may be disturbed by the trauma leading to avascular necrosis. The main supply penetrates the head close to the cartilage margin and arises from an arterial ring which feeds from the lateral and medial femoral circumflex arteries.

2. The head fragment is often a shell containing fragile spongy bone, and affords poor anchorage for any fixation device. Inadequate fixation may lead to non union.

Treatment. Preliminary skin traction to help relieve initial pain and minimize further displacement of the fracture. Analgesics should be appropriate to the patient's pain. However, through surgical treatment – generally by **open reduction internal fixation (ORIF)** – in some cases the patient may be mobilized as quickly as possible.

Intracapsular Fractures

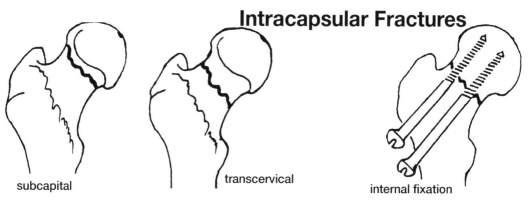

subcapital

transcervical

internal fixation

Mid Shaft Fracture of the Femur

Considerable trauma is usually required to fracture the femur, and the common causes include road traffic accidents, falls from heights and crushing injuries. Pathological fractures may also occur. With this kind of trauma, weight bearing is impossible and there is abnormal mobility in the limb at the level of the fracture. The leg is often externally rotated.

Treatment. Femoral shaft fractures are frequently treated conservatively and the first principle to appreciate is that the large muscle masses of the quadriceps and hamstrings tend to produce displacement and shortening. Traction can overcome this, and is the basis of most conservative methods of treatment. There are two methods of applying traction: **skin** or **skeletal** traction. The **Thomas splint** is normally used with this type of traction. It is fixed with a Pearson knee flexion piece. There are a few complications regarding a fracture of the femur, i.e. fat embolism, delayed union, non union, mal union and knee stiffness.

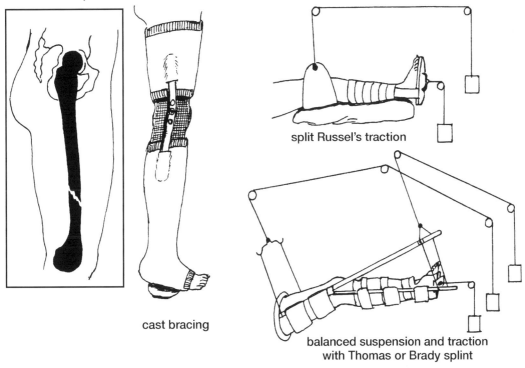

cast bracing

split Russel's traction

balanced suspension and traction
with Thomas or Brady splint

149

Supracondylar Fracture of the Femur

In children, fractures in the distal third of the femur are frequently only minimally displaced, and may be successfully treated by the application of a cylinder cast (stove pipe cast). Weight bearing should not be permitted till evidence of early union appears on the radiographs, but during this period the patient may be mobilized with crutches. In adults, supracondylar fractures have a strong tendency for the distal fragment to rotate under the continuous pull of the **gastrocnemius angulation** (anterior tilting). This cannot be controlled by traction in the line of the limb. It is necessary to flex the knee and maintain the traction over a fulcrum. The necessary degree of knee flexion may be obtained using a Pearson knee flexion piece, or better still by bending the Thomas splint at the level of the fracture. Mobilization of the knee should be started as early as possible as there is a high risk of knee stiffness from the development of tethering adhesions (between the quadriceps muscles and the hamstrings).

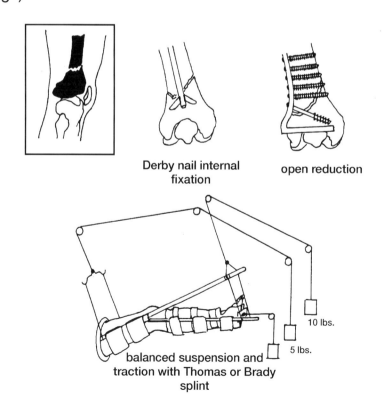

Derby nail internal
fixation

open reduction

balanced suspension and
traction with Thomas or Brady
splint

10 lbs.

5 lbs.

Fracture of the Patella

The patella may be fractured by direct trauma, as in a traffic accident in which the knee strikes the fascia or by a fall against a hard surface such as the edge of a step, or indirectly, as the result of a sudden muscle contraction. The same mechanism may also cause a rupture of the quadriceps tendon, rupture of the patella ligament or avulsion of the tibial tubercle. In most cases where there is a suspected fracture of the patella, extension of the knee will be difficult. If there are no other injuries, treatment is quite simple: six weeks in a cylinder (stove pipe) cast is usually adequate. The knee is normally kept in full extension but not in hyperextension (genu recuvartum), and crutches are usually avoided for the first two weeks.

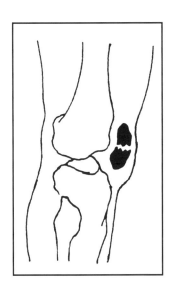

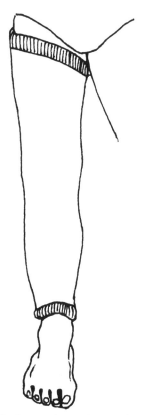

Cylinder or stove pipe cast

Ligamentous Injuries of the Knee

Knee joint instability may occur with the rupture of one or more of the supporting joints ligaments. The sensation of a joint "giving way" may be associated with supporting ligaments rupture. Take note that the knee is the largest joint in the body but not the strongest. The anterior and posterior **cruciate ligaments**, the medial and lateral **collateral ligaments**, and the **joint capsule** all work together to maintain the integrity of the knee. Twisting injuries, particularly those sustained during athletics, may sprain or rupture these ligaments to produce painful and often disabling conditions of the joint. Anterior cruciate ligament injuries will be frequently accompanied by rupture of the medial collateral ligament (MCL) and tears of the medial meniscus (attached to MCL). This combination is caused by severe trauma and is known as the **Terrible Triad**. After the operation, if the patient ends up with a **long-leg non walking cast (LLNW)** instead of a **continuous path of motion cast (CPM)**, the knee should be in at least 60° flexion and the foot in inversion in order to rest the ligaments. Make sure there is enough padding on the bony prominence area to avoid pressure (skin and nerve).

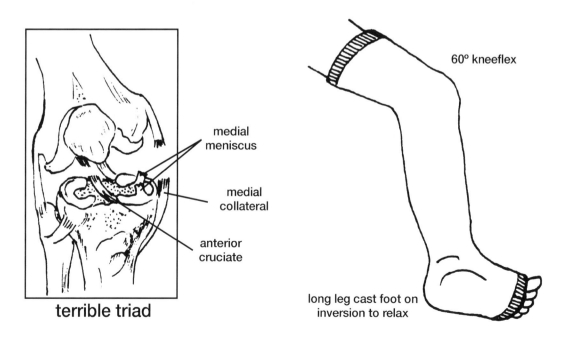

medial meniscus

medial collateral

anterior cruciate

terrible triad

60° kneeflex

long leg cast foot on inversion to relax

Tibial Fracture (Proximal)

Fractures of the upper end of the tibia may occur separately or in association, either with a fracture of the fibula just below the head, or dislocation outwards of that bone from the external tuberosity of the tibia. In all, the knee joint is implicated by the fracture so that there is hemorrhage of greater or lesser extent into the joint. In addition there is swelling and preternatural movement of the leg, which may even appear dislocated.

Treatment. In treating a fracture of the upper end of the tibia, the conditions of the ligaments, especially the cruciate, should be investigated, not so much as a guide to treatment, but for prognosis, since if there is marked antero-posterior movement of the tibia upon the femur, the result will be an unstable condition of the knee joint. If there is very little displacement, the extended leg should be put in plaster (LLNW) for about four weeks; however, if the joint alignment is poor an attempt should be made to correct it. The cast should remain on for four weeks, after which the patient may commence to move the knee and gradually restore movement. As soon as weight bearing is possible, the patient is allowed up on crutches. There is no difficulty about non-union in these fractures.

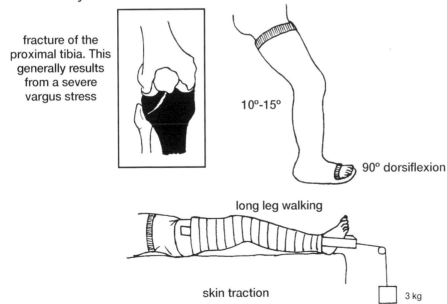

fracture of the proximal tibia. This generally results from a severe vargus stress

10°-15°

90° dorsiflexion

long leg walking

skin traction

3 kg

Tibial Fracture (Mid-Shaft)

The tibia is vulnerable to torsional stresses, to trauma transmitted through the feet and from direct blows. Note that a third of the tibia is subcutaneous. There is little to resist the spiky end of a fractured tibia from penetrating the skin. Again, any direct trauma to the shin is uncushioned, and the skin is readily split. These factors account for the frequency of both types of compounding in tibial shaft fractures. Partly because of the frequency of injury caused by torsional forces, oblique and spiral fractures of the tibia are common. Muscle tone in the **soleus, gastrocnemius** and **tibialis anterior** tends to produce shortening and displacement in fractures of this type.

Treatment. If the fracture is minimally displaced a long leg plaster is applied. Check radiographs for alignment. The limb should be elevated for 3 to 7 days until swelling subsides. The plaster is checked for slackness and changed if required. As soon as the patient has mastered crutches he may be allowed home. A walking heel is applied after 3 to 6 weeks, depending how much new bone development has occurred. The plaster is then retained until union. For early knee joint mobility there is an alternative depending on the union after 4 to 6 weeks post injury. The long leg cast is removed and a **Sarmiento** cast with a high condylar wing is applied. The plaster is retained until union is sound.

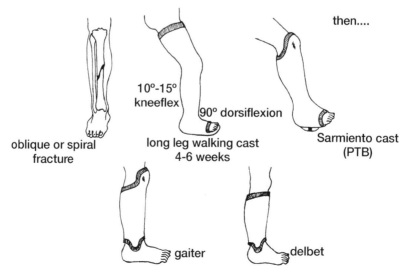

then....

10°-15° kneeflex

90° dorsiflexion

oblique or spiral fracture

long leg walking cast 4-6 weeks

Sarmiento cast (PTB)

gaiter

delbet

Tibial Fracture (Distal)

The function of the **ankle mortise** is threatened if the **malleoli** are fractured or the **tibiofibular** ligaments are torn. The stability of the **talus** may also be reduced by rupture of the medial or lateral ligaments. The most common injury is when the talus is rotated in the mortise, fracturing one or both malleoli. The classification of ankle fractures involving the ankle joint are often loosely referred to as **Pott's fractures**. In a first degree Pott's fracture, one malleoli is fractured. In a second degree Pott's fracture, two malleoli are fractured (bimalleolar fracture) and in a third degree Pott's fracture there is a bimalleolar fracture with an additional fracture of the posterior part of the inferior articular surface of the tibia (often referred to a the third malleolus). These fractures may also be referred to as **trimalleolar fractures**.

Treatment. The principles of treatment are to restore and maintain normal alignment of the talus with the tibia, creating good conditions for union or repair in the injured structures to ensure future stability and restore articulating surfaces to lessen the chances of osteoarthritis in the joint. Excellent results can be obtained by conservative treatment with below knee plasters or long leg plasters, depending on the severity of the trauma. Results are almost universally good; however, in a number of fractures, especially where there has been soft tissue interposition, reduction can only be achieved by open methods.

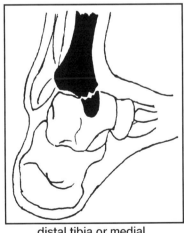

distal tibia or medial malleolus

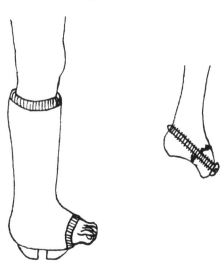

Tarsal Fracture

The talus plays a key role in no less than three joints: the ankle joint (articulating with the tibia and fibula), the subtalar joint (articulating with the calcaneus or os calcis), and the talonavicular joint, along with the calcaneoucuboid joint which forms the midtarsal joint. The common mechanism of injury for this type of fracture (neck of the talus) is the **Aviator Astragalus** type which occurs following a fall from a height in a crouching position. Complications for this fracture will be secondary osteoarthritis, perhaps followed by avascular necrosis. Take note that the blood supply of the talus enters at three sites: the neck, the sinus tarsi area and the medial side of the body. The more sources which are disturbed, the greater the risk to the blood supply. Conservative treatment for a type 1 injury should be a **below knee, non walking (BKNW)** plaster with toe platform, the foot plantar flexed and everted. If a satisfactory reduction has been obtained, then conservative treatment may be continued.

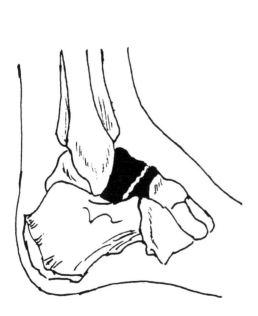

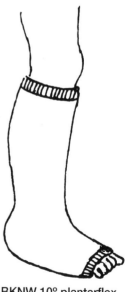

BKNW 10° plantarflex

Metatarsal Fracture

According to Ronald McRae (Practical Fracture Treatment, 1989), the most common fracture of the lower limb is an **avulsion** fracture of the base of the fifth metatarsal, following a sudden inversion strain. In an effort to correct the progressive inversion of the foot, the **peronei** contract violently and the **peroneus brevis** avulses its bony attachment.

Treatment. Most fractures are undisplaced but even marked displacement does not merit reduction if symptoms are slight. Apply a tensor or similar support for 2 to 3 weeks, and, if marked, a walking plaster for 5 to 7 weeks. Pain from the occasional non-union may be expected to resolve spontaneously, but Sudeck's atrophy is common and may require prolonged treatment. A **Jones fracture** (base of the fifth metatarsal) is not associated with inversion injuries, but tends to occur in athletes during training. Non-union is common, and is most often associated with early weight bearing. A **March** fracture is a fatigue fracture usually of the second metatarsal neck or shaft. This is not often seen until callus formation has occurred. If seen at an early stage, severe pain will occasionally merit treatment in a below knee walking plaster until union has taken place (2 to 3 weeks).

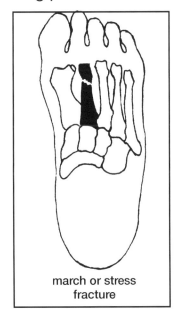

march or stress
fracture

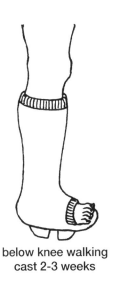

below knee walking
cast 2-3 weeks

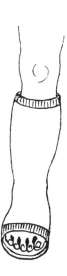

NOTES

CHAPTER 9
TRACTION GUIDELINES

General Information on Traction and Balanced Suspension

The purpose of any traction setup is one or more of the following:

- To prevent or reduce muscle spasm.
- To immobilize a joint or part of the body.
- To reduce a fracture or dislocation.
- To treat joint pathology(s).

It is important for the nurse/technician to know the patient's diagnosis so that an evaluation of the purpose and effectiveness of the apparatus can be made and, therefore, maintain the traction in such a way that its purpose is accomplished. To achieve these purposes, the traction setup must:

- Align the distal fragment to the proximal fragment.
- Remain constant.
- Allow for adequate exercise and diversion.
- Allow for optimum nursing care.

Traction and suspension setups are arrangements of bars, pulleys, ropes, and weights which exert a pulling force on a part or parts of the body, or serve to suspend or "float" a part of the body – most frequently a limb. The terms **traction** and/or **suspension** are often confused and used incorrectly or interchangeably. Many traction setups also include suspension; therefore, it is important for the nurse/technician to carefully study a particular setup to determine whether it is a traction, a suspension, or a combination of the two.

ANATOMICAL CONSIDERATIONS

Traction is the application of a pulling force to a part of the body. In order to fully understand this definition, a few basic anatomical facts about the human body must be considered.

The skeletal system **(see Chapter 2)** is composed of over 200 bones and is held in place by ligaments and muscles. These skeletal muscles act as "movers" of bones. A muscle group usually originates on one bone and terminates on another. Skeletal muscles have a tendon at each end which attach like strips of adhesive tape to the bone. When the brain signals a muscle to shorten (contract), the tendons at each end are pulled toward the center (belly) of the muscle. This exerts a force on the bones at each end of the muscle, and the bony part with the least resistance moves. Skeletal muscles have **tone**, which could be described as a state of readiness. Tone is continually producing a certain amount of pull on the tendons.

Figure 1 illustrates a broken femur. Notice the muscle groups have pulled the broken parts out of alignment. Proper traction and suspension will help restore position. The pull of the muscle group is overcome by a new force (traction) created with weights and pulleys.

Weights provide a constant (isotonic) force; pulleys help establish and maintain constant direction. The forces thus applied must remain constant in amount and direction until the fracture fragments unite.

Figure 2 illustrates the same femur after traction has been applied to realign (approximately) the broken parts. During an extensive period of healing, the limb must be supported to assist in maintaining fragment alignment, but the patient should still be able to move about as much as possible until union is achieved. This is why a second system of weights and pulleys called "balanced suspension" permits the limb to "float" over the bed and facilitates bedpan use and changing of bed linen with minimal disturbance of the fracture.

With all traction arrangements, countertraction is a consideration. Countertraction, which is the resistance of the body to move in the direction of the forces exerted by a traction device, is a factor which is built into each setup by utilizing the patient's body weight. When necessary, the countertraction of the patient's body weight may be increased by elevation of the foot of the bed or using blanket rolls, sand bags, etc.

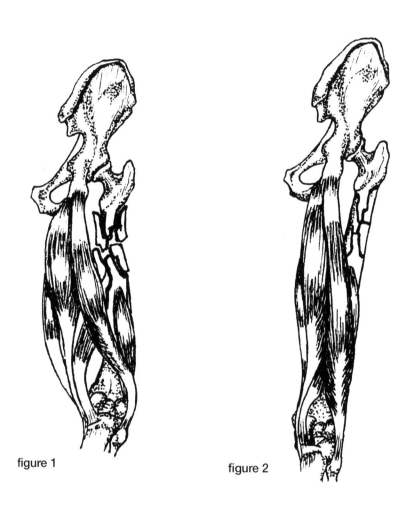

figure 1

figure 2

Types of Traction

There are three basic types of traction: **manual, skin** and **skeletal**. Each has its own special function in the management of fractures depending on physician preference, the type of fracture, and, in some cases, the patient herself.

☞ MANUAL TRACTION

In manual traction, the hands are used to exert a pulling force on the bone which is to be realigned **(Figure 3)**. Generally, this type of traction is reserved for very stable fractures or dislocations prior to splinting or immobilization in a cast. It may also be used prior to the application of skin or skeletal traction, or surgical reduction.

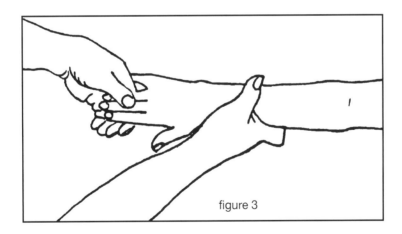

figure 3

☞ SKIN TRACTION

Strips of tape, moleskin, or some other type of commercial skin traction strips such as *Skin-Trac*® are applied directly to the skin **(Figure 4)**. Traction boots for leg traction and pelvic belts for spinal disorders also can be classified under this category.

The prime indication for skin traction is in the treatment of children's fractures and adult fractures or dislocations which require only a moderate amount of pulling force for a relatively short period. Certain types of children's fractures heal in a comparatively short time and do not require extremely heavy tractive forces to maintain bone alignment. Hence, the child's skin is more able to tolerate this type of traction than the adult's.

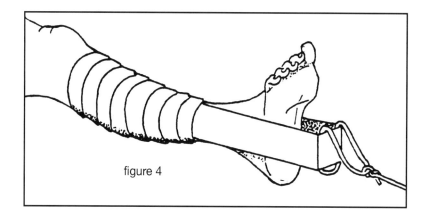

figure 4

For adults, skin traction is often used as a temporary measure prior to more definitive treatment such as open reduction or skeletal traction. Because of the possibility of severe skin irritation, skin traction should not be used on fractures which require more than 5 to 7 points of longitudinal force. It is also not recommended for continuous traction which is expected to exceed 3 to 4 weeks. Finally, skin traction is not recommended when controlling limb rotation of major importance.

☞ SKELETAL TRACTION

The tractive force is applied directly to the bone using pins, wires, screws, and, in the case of cervical traction, tongs applied directly to the skull. Skeletal traction allows the use of up to 20 or 30 pounds of force for as long as 3 to 4 months, if necessary. Moreover, it not only exerts a longitudinal pull, but also controls rotation.

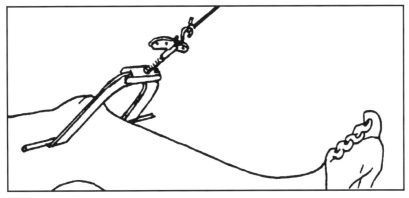
figure 5

Skeletal traction is particularly advantageous for unstable or fragmented fractures and those in which muscle forces must be overcome to maintain fracture alignment, e.g. fractures of the femoral shaft **(Figure 5)**.

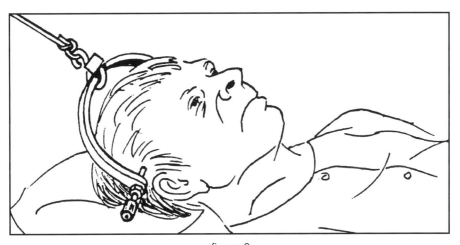
figure 6

For serious cervical spine fractures or injuries, Crutchfield, Vinke, or GardnerWells tongs are inserted directly into the skull and attached to the traction system. This stabilizes the vertebrae and reduces the chances of spinal cord damage or further injury **(Figure 6)**.

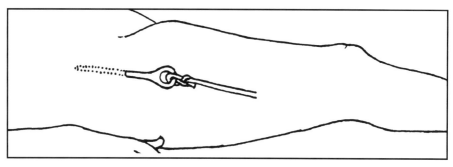

figure 7

For some fractures of the pelvis, a special pelvic traction screw is inserted into the ilium and connected to the traction system at the appropriate angle for maintaining fracture alignment **(Figure 7)**.

For long bone fractures, skeletal traction requires the use of Steinmann pins or Kirschner wires. The basic difference between the two is their diameter. Steinmann pins have a larger diameter, generally from 5/6" to 3/16" (2.0 mm to 4.8 mm). Kirschner wires generally range from .028" to 0.62" (.7 mm to 1.6 mm in diameter). Both pins also come in a variety of lengths and point styles **(Figure 8)**. These choices are generally based on physician preference, the density of bone through which the pin or wire is to be inserted, and the forces to be applied.

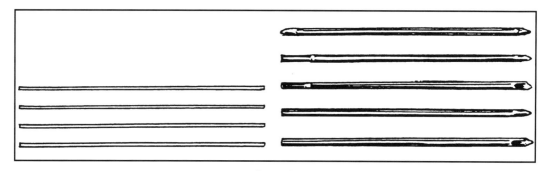

figure 8

Once inserted, the Steinmann pin or Kirschner wire is connected to its respective holder **(Figures 9, 10)**. The holder is then connected to the traction force. It must be emphasized that Steinmann pins are not compatible with the Kirschner Wire Tractor and vice versa. The Kirschner Wire Tractor and the Böhler Steinmann Pin Holder are designed for use only with their respective pins.

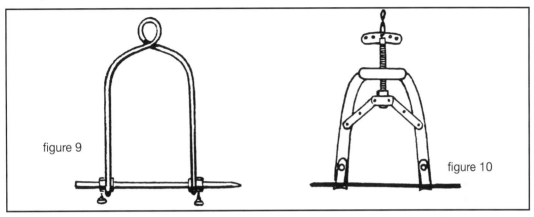

figure 9

figure 10

In addition to the previous classifications, traction also can be divided into two other categories based on the direction of force.

The first of these, straightline traction, is best exemplified by Buck's traction **(Figure 11)**. Here the traction is affixed to the limb at one point and then, using one or more pulleys, is attached to the weight. This causes the force to be applied in only one direction. Any change in the amount of applied force is the result of loss through friction caused by bedclothes, turning of pulleys, etc. Generally, any loss is negligible and, therefore, for each pound of weight applied, one (1) pound of force is delivered.

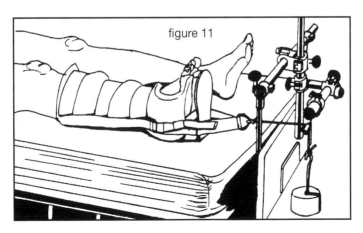

figure 11

The second category is the **block and tackle** or **suspensory** type of traction. Here, the traction system is attached to the patient in two or more places and also to one or more other stationary points on the traction frame. Each time the traction force is attached from the patient to the frame and back to the patient, directional lines of pull, or vectors of force, are being applied. Without applying complex mathematical equations, assume that for each time the body is attached to a pulley under continuous traction, the weight being applied increases by the number of attachments made. As an example, a 5-lb. weight will deliver approximately 15 lbs. of force on the femur **(Figure 12)**.

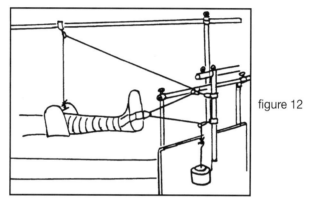

figure 12

The **vectors of force** principle is demonstrated with Russell's traction. As shown in **Figure 13**, the vertical pull on the sling (A-B) and the horizontal pull on the footplate (A-C) create a third force (A-D), along the axis of the femur. This is referred to as the **resultant force**. Any two or more forces acting on a body and not exactly opposed are known as vectors of force.

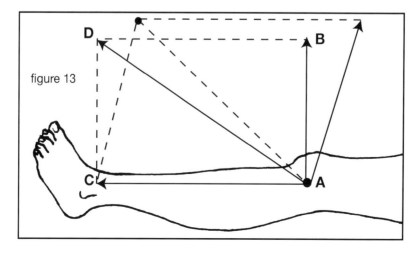

figure 13

Application of Traction

GENERAL TIPS AND PRECAUTIONS

Before you begin applying traction, remember:

☞ Skin traction cannot be applied over an open wound.

☞ Check with patient for possible adhesive allergies.

☞ **Do not reuse traction cord.** It does become worn and may eventually break. It can also become contaminated by bacteria.

After the above procedures have been completed, before threading the traction cord, lubricate all pulleys with silicone spray or a small amount of mineral oil. **Caution:** Never lubricate pulleys when traction is completely set up unless the attending physician is present to readjust the amount of weight. Lubrication changes the friction which, in turn, alters the balancing forces.

A concentrated effort should be directed towards avoiding pressure in the following locations:

Upper Extremities
*   Bony prominences about the elbow.
*   Anterior soft tissues of elbow joint.
*   Bony prominences about the wrist.

Lower Extremities
*   Peroneal nerves at the neck of the fibula.
*   Hamstring tendons at the back of the knee.
*   Bony prominences about the ankle.
*   Back of heels.
*   Soft tissues at front of ankle and top of foot.
*   Greater trochanters (outer area of upper thighs).

Trunk
- Prominences of spine.
- Borders of scapulae (shoulder blades).
- Crest of ilium (upper edges of pelvic bones).
- Sacral areas (tail bone).

Pressure on the elbow joints, wrists, knees and heels may be minimized by a generous wrapping of wide sheet wadding in order to distribute the weight of a limb over a wide area. Elevation of the ankle may be necessary to lift the tip of the heel away from the bed. PREVENTING A PRESSURE SORE IS EASIER THAN CURING ONE.

WEIGHTS

- Never add or remove weights without specific orders from the attending physician.

- Never allow weights to touch floor, drag on bed parts, or touch other weight systems. KEEP ALL WEIGHTS HANGING FREE.

- Do not allow traction weights to hang over any part of the patient. Traction cord does occasionally slip or break. If necessary, on some older types of apparatus, add an extra bar and pulley to get the weight in a freehanging position AWAY from the patient.

- Although the drawings in this handbook show the traction weights off the foot of the bed, some hospitals and physicians may require them to come off at the head of the bed. Both methods are acceptable; however, the reasoning behind each differs.

     From foot end:
1. Weights are out of patient's reach.
2. They are readily visible for inspection.
3. With shock blocks under the head of the bed, weights hang freely with less equipment.

From head of bed:
1. Weights are away from visitors' reach.
2. They are less subject to bumping by attending personnel.
3. Less equipment is required if shock blocks are under foot of bed.

•   Never apply pillows, sandbags, ice bags, hot water bottles, surgical dressings, cotton, sponge rubber, towels, felt, or any other type of pad to a patient in traction unless specifically ordered by the attending physician.

•   A routine should be established and followed to check each traction setup in detail. In addition, all nursing personnel coming into the patient's room should, out of habit, make a quick visual inspection of the equipment. This inspection should begin with the weights and follow along each rope to the patient to be sure that:
1. Weights are hanging free.
2. Ropes are in the pulleys, footplates, and spreader blocks.
3. Knots are free from pulleys.
4. Bed linens, etc., are not interfering with the traction forces.

Principles of Traction

RELATIONSHIP TO NURSING CARE

A great deal of the nursing care (and a good deal of equipment maintenance) related to the patient in any traction application is based upon certain principles. It is, therefore, imperative that the health care professional be constantly alert for the following:

☞ **POSITION:** The patient should be in the supine position (on her back). Proper position includes keeping the entire body in good alignment. Also, either a solid bottom bed or bed boards must be used for all orthopedic patients.

☞ **COUNTERTRACTION:** For any traction to be effective, there must be countertraction. If the force of pull of the traction is greater than the countertraction supplied by the body weight, the patient will slide towards the traction force, or the traction splint may impinge on the traction pulley. Should this happen, additional countertraction may be obtained by tilting the bed away from the traction force. Traction and countertraction represent forces in balance; for this reason the patient should not have his back raised more than 20°, or be allowed to sit up.

☞ **FRICTION:** Any type of friction will reduce the efficiency of traction and hinder the pull. Implications for nursing care include checking to see that:

a)   The spreader or footplate is not touching the end of the bed.

b)   The weights are positioned at a reasonable level from the floor; a considerable distance below the pulley; hanging free of the bed and away from the patient.

c)   There is no impingement on the traction cord from bedclothes or any other apparatus.

d)   The patient's heels are not digging into the mattress.

If any of these conditions are not being met, immediate corrective action is indicated.

☞ **CONTINUOUS:** In general, for traction to be effective, it must be continuous. NEVER remove it without a doctor's order. Furthermore, check frequently to make sure tapes are not slipping, and that pulleys are working properly.

☞ **LINE OF PULL:** Once established correctly, the line of pull should be maintained.

☞ **NEUROVASCULAR STATUS:** This should be checked every two hours. Check for skin color, sensation, temperature, motion and pulse. Any change from normal requires immediate attention.

☞ **SKIN EXAMINATION:** All skin traction systems require that skin checks be made routinely by removing elastic bandages, traction boots, etc. Manual traction should be maintained on the extremity during these checks to maintain alignment.

☞ **PATIENT SELF HELP:** Patients should be encouraged to help with their own care as much as possible. This will help them to maintain muscle tone, enhance circulation and contribute to their feeling of well-being.

☞ **NEVER IGNORE A PATIENT'S COMPLAINT:** This rule should be followed above everything else.

☞ **TRACTION SYSTEMS CAN VARY:** While it is essential for those caring for traction patients to know the correct application of traction, the nurse in change must remember that doctors may vary their traction methods for specific reasons. The nurse should, therefore, inform all floor personnel concerning any modifications to a particular traction setup instituted by a physician.

How to tie a Traction Knot

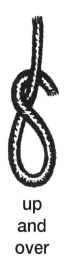
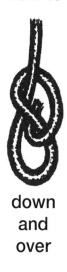
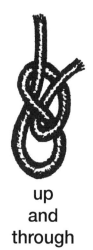
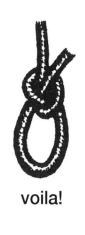

up
and
over

down
and
over

up
and
through

voila!

To save time, follow this simple phrase:

Up and Over, Down and Over, Up and Through.

Practice a few times with a traction cord and this illustration. It is a good idea to secure all knots tightly with adhesive tape.

Contraindications to Skin Traction

1. Abrasions of the skin (scraping away a portion of skin)

2. Lacerations of the skin in the area to which the traction is to be applied (a wound or irregular tear of the flesh)

3. Impairment of circulation – varicose ulcers, impending gangrene

4. Dermatitis – inflammation of skin

5. Marked shortening of the bony fragments, when the traction weight required will be greater than can be applied through the skin.

Complications of Skin Traction

1. Allergic reactions to the adhesive.

2. Excoriation of the skin from slipping of the adhesive strapping (abrasion of the epidermis).

3. Pressure sores around the malleoli and over the tendo calcaneus.

4. Common peroneal nerve palsy. This may result from two causes: Rotation of the limb is difficult to control with skin traction. There is a tendency for the limb to rotate laterally and for the common peroneal nerve to be compressed by the slings on which the limb rests. Also, adhesive strapping tends to slide slowly down the limb, carrying the encircling bandage with it. The circumference of the limb around the knee is greater than that around the head of the fibula. The downward slide of the adhesive strapping and bandages may be halted at the head of the fibula, which can cause pressure on the common peroneal nerve.

Complications of Skeletal Traction

1. Introduction of infection into bone.

2. Incorrect placement of the pin or wire may:
    -   allow the pin or wire to cut out of the bone and cause the failure of the traction system
    -   make control of rotation of the limb difficult
    -   make the application of splint difficult
    -   result in an uneven pull being applied to the ends of the pin or wire and thus cause the pin or wire to move in the bone. This movement will result in an increased risk of infection in the bone and ischaemic necrosis of the skin around the pin or wire from pressure on the skin by the Böhler stirrup or Kirschner wire strainer (yoke/bow)

3. Distraction at the fracture site as very large traction forces can be applied through skeletal traction.

4. Ligamentous damage if a large traction force is applied through a joint for a prolonged period of time.

5. Damage to epiphyseal growth plates when used in children. **Genu recurvatum** can occur as a late complication of the treatment of a fracture of the femoral shaft in children with traction through the upper end of the tibia.

6. Depressed scars: These can be prevented if the pin track is pinched at the time of removal of the pin, to rupture the bridge of fibrous tissue which forms between the skin and periosteum.

Bradford Frame and Thomas Splint

Indications. For a patient with a fractured femur. Used for toddler to pre-teen patient.

Position of bed and patient. The frame is hooked at the end of the bed in a 45° angle. The patient should lie flat on back with no pillow. Countertraction may be increased by elevating foot of bed with bed blocks. Physician may alter the traction.

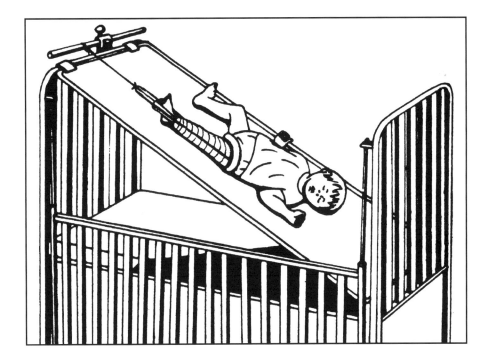

Tips and Precautions.

- Neurovascular signs should be checked every 2 to 4 hours.

- Check skin for any irritation or allergic reaction to the traction tapes.

- Thomas splint should be sized for the patient and should be long enough to allow him/her to plantarflex and dorsiflex foot.

- The ring of the Thomas splint should be well up in the groin without restricting circulation or causing the patient any discomfort. The caregiver should be able to put two fingers between ring and groin.

- When assessing a patient in a Thomas splint, one should check for the following:

❑ Make sure splint is secure to the end of the bed.
❑ Leg should be in a functional position.
❑ Make sure the ankle area is well padded to prevent any pressure sores.
❑ Check flannel bandages to make sure they are not too snug.
❑ Check traction tapes for slipping (tapes are usually marked for each assessment).
❑ Make sure the proximal and distal leg is supported. The heel should be free to avoid pressure sores from developing.
❑ Check ring of the splint to make sure it is not restricting circulation. You should be able to insert at least one finger between limb and ring.
❑ Patient should not have a pillow or be sitting, unless doctor orders.

- Encourage patient to be independent.

- Encourage passive and active exercises of foot.

- Bradford frame (bed linen) should be changed daily.

Choosing a Thomas splint. Measure to oblique circumference of thigh immediately below the **gluteal fold** and **ischial tuberosity.** This measurement equals the internal circumference of the ring. Add 1" to 2" to allow for swelling. Measure the distance from the crotch to the heel and add 6" to 9" to allow patient to dorsiflex and plantarflex foot. Measurement should be done medially.

Traction set-up.
1   Bradford frame (sized according to patient)
1   Hook
1   Thomas splint (sized for patient)
2   Extension traction tapes
2   Rolls of flannel bandages
     Silence cloths
     Factory cloths
     Rope
     Webbing tape, 18"

The Thomas splint should be secured at the end of the bed.

Changing tapes.

- Apply tincture of benzoin on limb.
- Using silence cloth, pad ankle area well.
- Apply traction tapes.
- Wrap limb with flannel bandages, leaving knee exposed.
- Secure to Thomas splint using webbing tape.
- Cradle leg using factory cloth for upper leg and silence cloth for lower leg.

Slings and Springs

Indications. These are indicated for patients with Legg Perthes disease, as well as for post-operative hip surgery for most patients over the age of seven (7) years. The patient should lie flat on his back with the affected leg in slings and springs. The head of the bed may be elevated for meals. This can be applied bilaterally. The reason for slings and springs is to allow a range of motion of the hip. Unless the patient is going for tests and physiotherapy, she should remain in the set-up at all times.

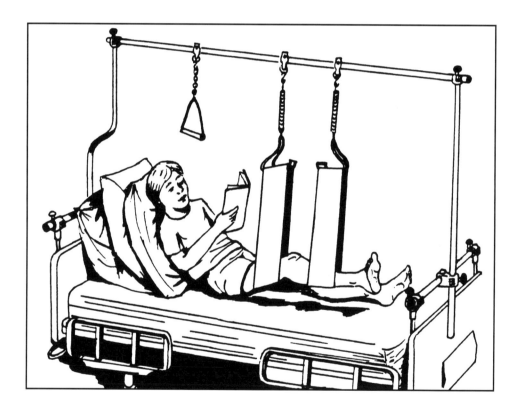

Tips and Precautions.

- The proximal sling should support the thigh without forcing the knee to flex; the leg should be in full extension.

- The distal sling should support the calf; the heel should be free to prevent any pressure sores.

- Very little complication can occur with this set-up, but one should check to make sure the proximal sling is not causing any pressure in the popliteal space.

- Encourage the patient to exercise and explain why it is important for him/her to do so.

- It is important for a patient with Legg Perthes not to weight-bear on the affected leg.

- Since most of these patients are not sick, they will need lots of diversion to keep them happy to remain in bed.

Gallows Traction (Bryant's)

Indications. This is indicated in fractures of the femur in children up to two years old or weighing less than 30 pounds (14 kg.), as well as for stabilization of the hip joint where use of the cast is not indicated.

General Information. Traction is bilateral (even if pathology is unilateral) to help prevent rotation and to facilitate better stabilization of the patient, thereby maintaining better control.

Position of bed and patient. With the bed in a level position and the patient flat on the bed, vertical suspension traction of the legs should be set up so that the hips are flexed at right angles. When the traction is in place, the buttocks should just clear the mattress. Lift the buttocks a few inches off the mattress. When the buttocks are released, the child should return to the "just clear" position described above. If not, check with the attending physician regarding a possible change in the amount of weight.

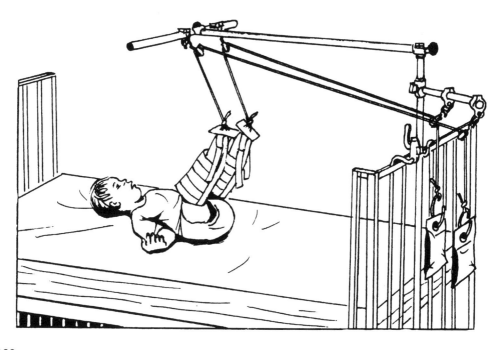

Tips and Precautions.

- **Warning:** Dangerous complications leading to ischemic contractures **CAN** occur. Check both feet at least every two hours for color, pulse, motion, temperature, and sensation.

- Check for undue pressure:
- a) Over the outer head and neck of the fibula.
- b) On the dorsum of the foot.
- c) On the Achilles tendon.

- Check to see that bandages, boots, etc. have not slipped and become bunched around the toes or ankles.

- Problems with this type of traction are difficult to define due to the age of the child. These problems include:
- 1. Inability to communicate wants and needs.
- 2. Toilet needs.
- 3. Feeding.
- 4. Diversion.
- 5. Maintaining position which makes it sometimes necessary to use some form of jacket or restraint, especially to keep the child from "rotating" around the traction apparatus.

- All of the above need to be handled with individual consideration. Get to know the child. Talk with the parents!

Cervical Traction

Indications. This form of traction is indicated for cervical myositis, dislocations, arthritis and/or degenerative spinal disorders and whiplash. It may also be indicated for minor fractures. (More serious fractures would be treated by skeletal traction, using Vinke, Crutchfield, or Gardner-Wells tongs).

Position of bed and patient. If possible, position the patient flat on back with the bed in the level position, unless otherwise prescribed by the physician. Additional countertraction may be accomplished by putting the head of the bed on elevation blocks, or by raising the backrest.

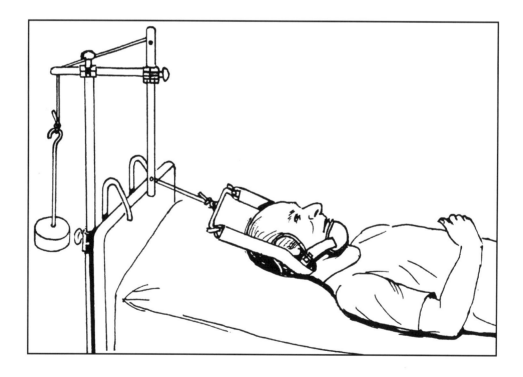

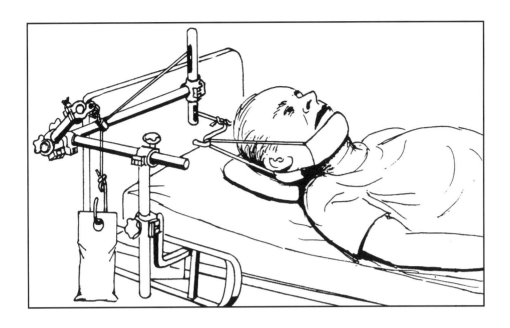

Tips and Precautions.

- Patient may be positioned with his or her head at the foot end of the bed when a Buck's extension bracket is used on certain types of beds.

- Hyperextension may be increased by placing a rolled towel or tension pillow beneath the patient's neck.

- Use a spreader bar which is wide enough so that the head halter does not touch the side of the patient's head or pinch his or her ears.

- Additional felt padding, frequent routine changing of the padding and cornstarch or powder will help reduce skin irritation.

- Due to the biomechanics of jaw loading, pain may develop in the ears or mandibular joint. A mouth guard, such as those used by athletes, may help relieve this problem.

- Occasionally, with permission from the attending physician, the patient may have the traction released for brief periods.

- Prism glasses can make watching TV or reading easier.

- Check occipital area for pressure spots. Patients in cervical traction can develop pressure sores in this area.

- Chewing and swallowing are frequently difficult. Diet modifications may be necessary to ensure adequate intake.

- Establish eye contact by standing where the patient can see you!

- Always remember to turn off the overhead lights when not needed. A light shining directly in a patient's eyes is irritating.

Traction on Humerus With Side Arm Frame

Indications. This type of traction is indicated in cases of immobilization or stabilization of fractures, dislocations and other pathology of the upper arm and shoulder. It is necessary to establish an angle of pull which produces the best possible alignment for reduction of the fracture.

Position of bed and patient. The patient should be flat on her back with the injured forearm flexed and extended 90° from, and in the same plane as, the upper body. The bed may be flat, or, if ordered by the physician, the backrest may be elevated.

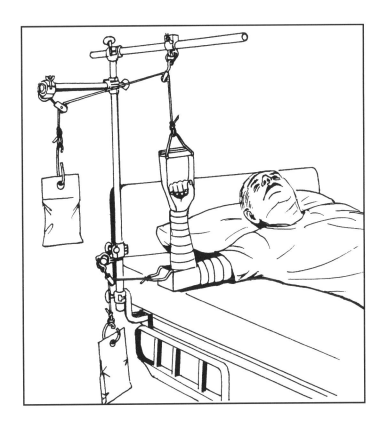

Tips and Precautions.

- Traction is applied to the humerus only. The forearm is only in balanced suspension.

- An overhead frame and trapeze will facilitate patient care and enable the patient to be more active and help himself.

- Exposed adhesive sides of SKIN-TRAC® traction strips should be covered near the hand and other bony prominences to prevent sticking and skin irritation.

- Countertraction can be increased by:
  a. Placing a rolled blanket between the mattress and spring on the traction side of the bed.
  b. Placing bed elevation or shock blocks under the bed on the traction side of the bed to tilt the patient away from the traction.
  c. Using a body or jacket restraint to keep the patient away from the traction side of the bed.

- Encourage active and passive exercises especially to the wrist and fingers of the affected arm.

- The bed linen is most easily changed from top to bottom.

- Make sure bandage wrappings are not tighter at the proximal rather than distal end of the arm; otherwise swelling may occur.

- Make sure wrapping bandages are not cutting at the elbow or wrist. This can be prevented by placing a piece of felt padding in these areas.

- Due to its elevated and immobile position, the hand may feel cold to the patient even though circulation is adequate. A light covering, such as a towel, can relieve this problem.

- Frequent and thorough back care is essential to prevent skin breakdown as well as to relieve the general discomfort resulting from remaining in the supine position for an extended period.

- Since the patient has the use of only one hand (and frequently not the one normally used), he or she may require help with eating to ensure adequate dietary and fluid intake. These patients also will need help with other self care procedures such as teeth brushing, hair combing, etc. Keep items such as water, tissues, etc. within easy reach.

- Remember to turn off overhead lights when not needed. A light shining directly in a patient's eyes is irritating.

- Patients in 90-90 traction will need prism glasses for reading and watching TV.

- Be sure to stand where the patient can see you!

Traction on Humerus-Overhead (90-90)

Indications: Indicated in cases of immobilization or stabilization of fractures, dislocations, and other pathology of the upper arm and shoulder. The establishment of an angle of pull is required in order to produce the best possible alignment for reduction of the fracture.

Position of bed and patient. If possible, the bed should be level with the patient flat on back.

Tips and Precautions. These are similar to those for the side arm frame.

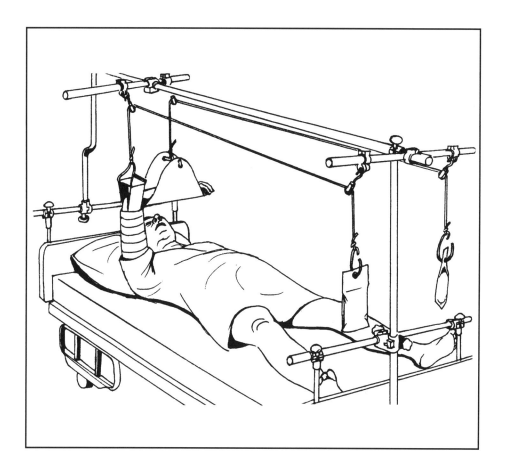

Pelvic Traction with Pelvic Belt

Indications. This is indicated in the following situations:
1. Trial treatment of nerve root disorders.
2. Sciatica.
3. Muscle spasms (low back).
4. Minor fractures of lower spine.

Position of bed and patient. The attending physician may prescribe countertraction either by:

1. Elevation of the foot of the bed using shock blocks;
2. Gatching of the bed at the knees;
3. Placing pillows under the knees, or
4. Placing the bed in the semiFowler's (jackknife) position.

Whichever countertraction the physician prescribes, the patient should be flat on her back.

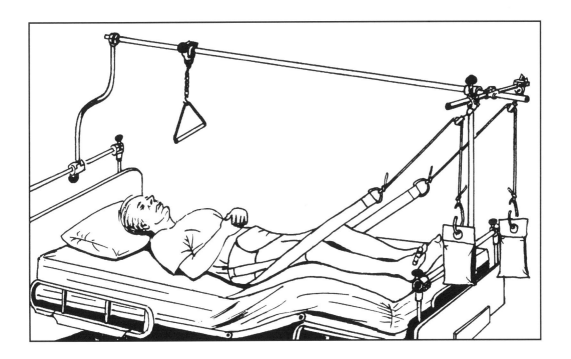

Tips and Precautions.

- Check and adjust pelvic belt straps so they are unrestricted and equal in length. It is a good idea to secure the straps with adhesive tape or a safety pin.

- Make sure the angle of pull is correct.

- Since the pelvic belt is applied directly to the skin, check frequently for skin irritation, especially on the iliac crests. Powder and other skin care measures can help prevent skin irritation and breakdown.

- Pelvic belts should be changed and laundered when they become soiled, or at least every three days.

- Constipation will add to patient discomfort. Measures should be taken to prevent this condition and patients should be taught why these measures are necessary.

- A footboard will help prevent foot drop.

- Back pain is often difficult to define and relieve, but it is very real. Moral support is essential for these patients. They also should be instructed on proper body mechanics and care of the back to prevent future disorders.

Traction setup.

1. Attach basic frame setup to bed.

2. Attach 36" (91 cm) center clamp bar to overhead bar at extreme foot end of bed. NOTE: One 9" (23 cm) single clamp bar may be placed on the upright bar at the foot of the bed for attachment of one 36" (91 cm) for attachment of one 36" (91 cm) center clamp bar to provide greater clearance for weights).

3.   Attach two pulleys to 36" (91 cm) center clamp bar.

4.   Measure the patient's girth at the crest of the ilium to insure correct size of belt.

5.   Apply pelvic traction so that the lower portion of the belt is at or slightly below the greater trochanter. (The belt is not to be applied like an abdominal binder.)

6.   Attach traction cords to straps of pelvic belt, thread through pulleys, then tie to weight carriers.

7.   Apply weights.

NOTE: The above procedure may be altered using a 22" (56 cm) spreader bar and a single traction cord, pulley, and weight carrier. The 36" (91 cm) center clamp bar can be deleted, and a 9" (23 cm) single clamp bar with pulley can be attached at an angle to the upright bar at the foot of the bed.

Buck's Unilateral Leg Traction (One Leg)

Indications. This is indicated in the following instances:
1.   Trial treatment of nerve root disorders.
2.   Sciatica.
3.   Muscle spasms
4.   Minor fractures of the lower spine.
5.   Temporary stabilization of fractured hips or fractures of the femoral shaft.
6.   Degenerative arthritis and knee injuries.

Position of bed and patient. The patient should be flat on his back with the foot of the bed elevated.

Tips and Precautions.

*   Pulley bars must be placed so that the line of pull aligns distal to proximal.

*   Cover exposed adhesive side of *Skin-Trac*® traction strips* (if used) near the angles with strips of felt or sheet wadding to prevent them from sticking to the foot and ankles.

*   Make sure wrappings are not too tight across the dorsum of the foot. Excess pressure can cause severe complications.

*   Pressure on the heels can cause irritation and skin breakdown. Make sure heels are not digging into the mattress. If necessary, place small foam pads, folded blankets, etc., under full length of the calf to keep heels off the bed.

*   Make sure pressure is kept off the peroneal nerve, or foot drop may occur.

*   A bed cradle may be used to keep bed covers from resting on the feet.

- Encourage activity as tolerated, including active and passive exercises. The patient should use the trapeze for moving about in bed.

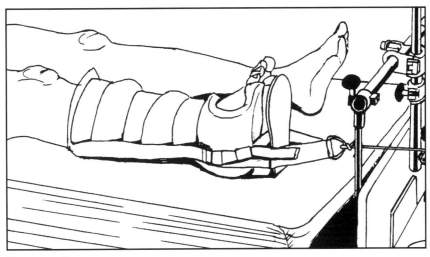

Traction setup.

1. Attach basic frame setup to bed.

2. Attach one 5" (13 cm) single clamp bar to upright bar at foot of bed. NOTE: A 9" (23 cm) single clamp may be used for greater clearance of the weights.

3. Attach one 9" (23 cm) single clamp bar to 5" (13 cm) single clamp bar.

4. Attach pulley to 9" (23 cm) single clamp bar.

5. Apply Deluxe Convoluted *Zim-Trac®* Perforated Traction Splint* to leg.

6. Tie traction cord to splint, thread through pulley, and then tie to weight carrier.

7. Apply weights.

NOTE: The above procedure may be altered by using *Skin-Trac®* Skin Traction Strips* wrapped with a *Zimmer®* Premium or Standard Orthopedic Wrap*.

Buck's Biilateral Leg Traction (Both Legs)

Indications. Indications are the same as for Buck's Unilateral Leg Traction.

Position of bed and patient. The patient should be flat on his back with the bed gatched at the knees. (The physician may prescribe elevation blocks as a means of additional countertraction.)

Traction setup.
1. Attach basic frame setup to bed.

2. Attach 5" (13 cm) single clamp bar to upright bar at foot of bed. NOTE: A 9" (23 cm) single clamp bar may be used for greater clearance of the weights.

3. Attach 36" (91 cm) center clamp bar to 5" (13 cm) single clamp bar.

4. Attach pulleys to 36" (91 cm) center clamp bar.

5. Apply Deluxe Convoluted *Zim-Trac*® Perforated Traction Splints* to legs.

6. Tie traction cord to splints, thread through pulleys, then to weight carriers.

7. Apply weights.

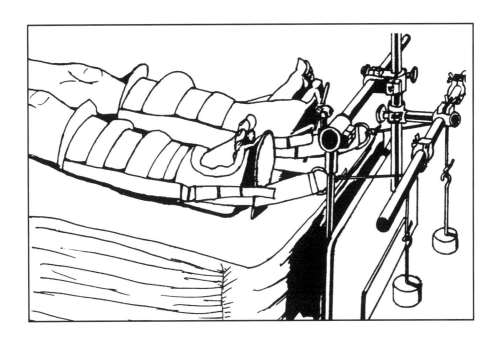

Unilateral Leg Traction Using Böhler-Braun Frame

Indications: This is indicated for comminuted fractures extending into the knee joint, unstable fractures of the tibia or femur, and open fractures associated with severe soft tissue damage. It can be applied with either skin or skeletal traction, and is especially useful for patients where transportation is necessary since the traction apparatus is self-contained.

Position of bed and patient. Patient should be flat on back with the bed level.

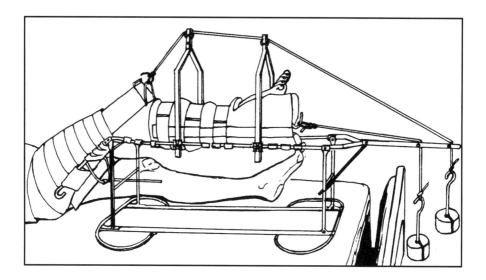

Tips and Precautions.

- Slings should be placed so no pressure is on the popliteal space, Achilles tendon, or the heel.

- Make sure elastic bandages are not tighter at the proximal rather than at the distal end of the femur and/or lower leg; otherwise swelling may occur.

- Make sure the proximal end of the frame does not press into the perineum. A large dressing or pieces of sheepskin can be used to pad this area and can be easily changed if soiled.

- An overhead frame and trapeze will allow the patient to move about more easily.

- Apply an anti-embolism stocking to the unaffected leg.

- Usually, the patient can turn upwards the splint for back care, linen changes, etc. It may be easier if the bed is made with two folded sheets, one at the head and another at the foot, underneath the splint. Then, if only one part of the bed needs changing, the splint will not have to be moved.

- Pressure from slings, wrappings, etc. or from the leg lying against the side of the frame can cause peroneal nerve damage. Make sure the leg is not externally rotated, and check the neurovascular status every two hours.

- If skeletal traction is used, refer to your institution's policies regarding care of the pin sites.

Traction setup

1. Attach canvas slings (provided) no frame.

2. Apply separate strips of *Skin-Trac*® Skin Traction Strips* smoothly to the upper or lower leg, according to the traction position prescribed by the attending physician. (If splint is for temporary stabilization only, application of skin traction may be eliminated in certain instances).

3. Wrap *Zimmer*® Premium or Standard Orthapaedic Wrap* around *Skin-Trac*® Skin Traction Strips* on the leg. NOTE: A Deluxe Convoluted *Skin-Trac*® Perforated Traction Splint* may be used on lower portion of leg in place of *Skin-Trac*® Skin Traction Strips and bandages.

4. Lift injured leg and place the frame under it with the knee directly over the angle of the frame.

5. Adjust the towers or sling so that any pressure points are eliminated. (Protect heel and hamstring tendons.)

6. Tie traction cord to spreader block and foot piece, thread through pulleys. Then tie to weight carriers.

7. Attach spreader block and foot piece to *Skin-Trac®* Skin Traction Strips.*

8. Apply weights.

Russel's Traction

Indications. This is indicated in the treatment of certain types of knee injuries, and for fractures of the shaft of the femur or hip.

Position of bed and patient. Proper countertraction is obtained either by elevating the foot of the bed, or by gatching the bed at the knees with the patient flat on his back. In certain instances, the head of the bed may be elevated, but only at the discretion of the attending physician. The physician may also order a pillow placed under the affected leg. If so, this must be checked frequently to make sure proper alignment is maintained.

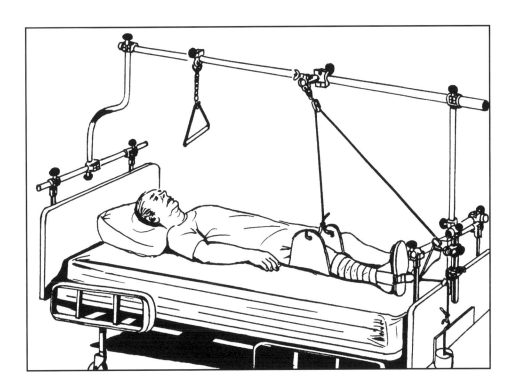

Tips and Precautions.

- Make certain that the knee sling is smooth and that its edges do not cut into the soft tissues.

- Due to the pulley arrangement, the pull on the foot is double that of the weight applied. **(See vectors of force)**.

- If a pillow is ordered for under the calf when the traction is initially set up, it must remain in place. Removing it can change the vectors of force and alignment.

- Arrangements of Russell's traction vary. Therefore, be aware of how it was set up initially.

- Nursing care is simplified by suspension of the limb, which allows the patient to lift and move about with minimal disturbance to the line of pull. This suspension is achieved through the delicate balance of traction and countertraction resulting from the distribution of weight through the various elements.

- Proper application of *Skin-Trac*® Skin Traction Strips* and wrapping of elastic bandages are crucial to the prevention of peroneal nerve damage. Neurovascular checks must be made at least every two hours.

- Active and passive exercises should be done routinely. The patient should be encouraged to do as much for herself as possible. Good skin care is also imperative.

- An anti-embolism stocking should be applied to the unaffected leg on all adult patients.

Split Russel's Traction

Indications. This is indicated for fractures of the femoral shaft, hip and lower leg or any combination of these, as well as for the treatment of certain types of knee injuries.

Position of bed and patient. Proper countertraction is obtained either by elevating the foot of the bed, or by gatching the bed at knees with the patient flat on his back. In certain instances, the head of the bed may be elevated, but only at the discretion of the attending physician. The physician may also order a pillow placed under the affected leg. If so, this must be checked frequently to make sure proper alignment is maintained.

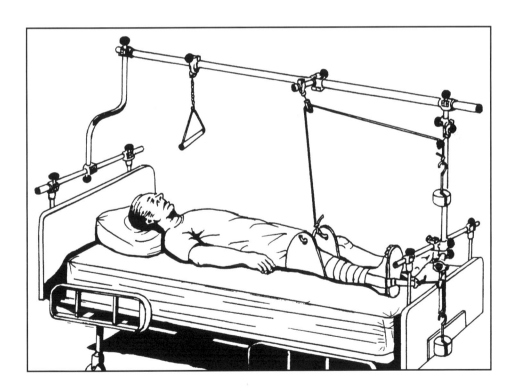

Balanced Suspension and Traction with Thomas or Brady Leg Splint (Using Skin or Skeletal Traction)

Indications. This is indicated for fractures of the femoral shaft hip, and lower leg, or any combination of these. The only basic difference between the Thomas and Brady systems is that the Brady system is universally sized, whereas the Thomas is sized to fit individual patients.

Position of bed and patient. Elevate the foot of the bed with the patient flat on her back. (In certain instances, the head of the bed may be elevated, but only at the discretion of the attending physician).

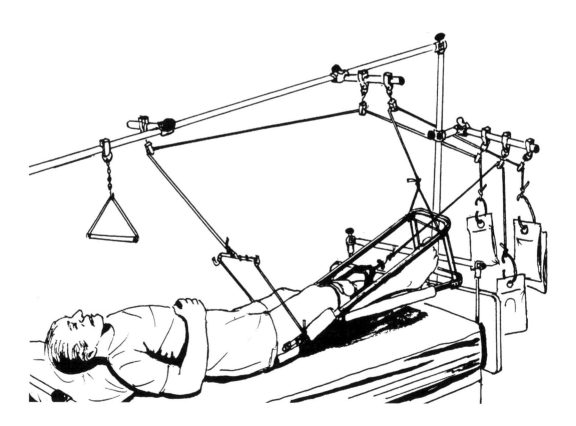

Tips and Precautions.

- Padding the ischial ring with sheepskin enhances patient comfort. The sheepskin can be easily removed when soiled without affecting the balance of the setup.

- Meticulous skin care and decubitus prevention measures must be carried out routinely.

- Active and passive exercises should be done at least four times a day.

- Make sure the leg does not rotate externally and place pressure on the peroneal nerve. Check the neurovascular status of the limb at least every two hours.

- If elastic bandages are used, they should be checked frequently for excessive pressure at the site of the fibular head and the dorsum of the foot.

- Slings should be positioned so that the heel and Achilles tendon do not carry the weight of the lower leg.

- Patients in this type of suspension and traction initially experience much discomfort and are very apprehensive. The nurse needs to explain all procedures as well as enlist the cooperation of the patient in helping with his or her care.

- The patient generally finds a fracture bedpan more convenient.

- It is easier to make the bed from the head to the foot. The patient can lift her head and shoulders by using the trapeze.

- In most cases, the patient should wear an anti-embolism stocking on the unaffected leg.

- For skeletal traction, refer to your own institution's policies regarding care of the pin site.

*Trademarks of Zimmer Orthopaedic Surgical Products Inc.

ROOTS

1. adeno .... gland
2. angio .... blood vessel
3. arterio .... artery
4. arthro .... joint
5. broncho .... bronchus (lower wind pipe)
6. cardio .... heart
7. cephalo .... head, brain
8. cranio .... head, brain
9. cysto .... sac, cyst, bladder
10. cyto .... cell
11. derma, dermato .... skin
12. entero .... intestines
13. fibro .... fibrons, fibres
14. gastro .... stomach
15. hem, hemato, hemo, hema .... blood
16. hystero .... uterus
17. laryngo .... larynx (voice box)
18. myelo .... bone marrow, spinal cord
19. myo .... muscle
20. nephro .... kidney
21. neuro .... nerve
22. oophoro .... ovary
23. ophthalmo .... eye
24. osteo .... bone
25. ovario .... ovary
26. phryngo .... pharynx
27. phlebo .... vein
28. pneumo .... lung, air
29. procto .... rectum
30. rhino .... nose
31. stoma .... mouth
32. thoraco .... chest, thorax
33. tracheo .... trachea (windpipe)
34. uro .... urine, urinary
35. veno .... vein

SUFFIXES

1. algia ....pain
2. cele ....protrusion
3. centesis...puncture
4. desis...fixation
5. ectasis...dilation
6. ectomy...removal of
7. genic...originating in
8. itis...inflammation of
9. lithotomy ....incision for removal of stones
10. lysis ....breaking down
11. megaly...enlargement
12. oid ....like
13. oma...tumor
14. oscopy ....inspection of
15. osis ....condition of disease
16. ostomy...creation of a permanent opening
17. otomy ....opening into
18. pathy..disease
19. penia..decrease
20. pexy...suspension, fixation
21. plasty ....repair
22. ptosis ....falling
23. rrhapy ....suture
24. spasm...involving prolonged contraction
25. rrhea ....flow
26. rrhagia ....excessive flow

References Cited and Bibliography

Adams, John Crawford, MD, MS, FRCS.
    1976 Outline of Orthopaedics, Eighth Edition. Churchill Livingstone.

Blauvelt, Carolyn Taliaferro and Nelson, Fred R. T., MD, FACS, FAAOS.
    1990 A Manual of Orthopaedic Terminology. C. V. Mosby.

Bleck, E. E., MD
    1974 Atlas of Plaster Cast Techniques, Second Edition.
    Yearbook Medical Publishers.

Blount, Walter Putnam, AB, MD, FACS.
    1955 Fractures in Children. Williams and Wilkins.

Brunner, Nancy A, RN, BSN.
    1970 Orthopaedic Nursing: A Programmed Approach. C. V. Mosby.

Duckworth, T., BSc, MB, ChB, FRCS.
    1984 Lecture Notes on Orthopaedics and Fractures.
    Blackwell Scientific Publications.

Gartland, John J., MD.
    1987 Fundamentals of Orthopaedics. W. B. Saunders.

Ginness, Alma E. (Ed.)
    1987 ABC's of the Human Body: A Family Answer Book.
    Readers' Digest

Gunn, Christine, TDCR
    1992 Bones and Joints: A Guide for Students, Second Edition.
    Churchill Livingstone.

Gustillo, Ramon B., MD.
    1991 The Fracture Classification Manual. C. V. Mosby.

Guy, Julia F, MS, PhD.
    1992 Learning Human Anatomy: A Laboratory Text and
    Workbook. Prentice Hall.

Howard, L. D.
    Casts: Things Heal Faster in Plaster.

McRae, Ronald, FRCS, AIMBI.
    1989 Practical Fracture Treatment. Churchill Livingstone.

Marieb, Elaine N., RN, PhD.
    1994 Essentials of Human Anatomy and Physiology,
    Fourth Edition. Benjamin Cummings.
    1992 Essentials of Human Anatomy and Physiology,
    Second Edition. Benjamin Cummings.

Salib, Philip I., MD, FACS
    1975 Plaster Casting. Prentice Hall.

Schade, MD, PhD.
    1970 Introduction to Functional Human Anatomy: An Atlas.
    W. B. Saunders.

Snell, Richard S., MD, PhD.
    1992 Clinical Anatomy for Medical Students, Fourth Edition.

Solomon, Eldra Pearl and Phillips, Gloria A.
    1987 Understanding Human Anatomy and Physiology.
    W. B. Saunders.

Stewart, John D. M., MA, FRCS, and Hallett, Jeffery P., MA, FRCS.
    1983 Traction and Orthopaedic Appliances. Churchill Livingstone.

Thibodeau, Gary A., PhD.
    Structure and Function of the Body.

Wilson, George Ewart, MB, ChB, FRCS.
    1930 Fractures and Their Complications. Macmillan.

Made in the USA
Columbia, SC
20 December 2020